Latest Advances in Cochlear Implant Technologies and Related Clinical Applications

Edited by Stavros Hatzopoulos, Andrea Ciorba and Piotr H. Skarzynski

Published in London, United Kingdom

Latest Advances in Cochlear Implant Technologies and Related Clinical Applications
http://dx.doi.org/10.5772/intechopen.105308
Edited by Stavros Hatzopoulos, Andrea Ciorba and Piotr H. Skarzynski

Contributors
Bettina Carvalho, Rogerio Hamerschmidt, Gislaine Richter Minhoto Wiemes, Nicole Richter Minhoto Wiemes, Maksym Situkho, Viktor Lutsenko, Yevhen Antonov, Viliam Dolinay, Liia V. Toropchina, Elena I. Zelikovich, Maria Lalayants, Isra Aljazeeri, Abdulrahman Hagr, Yassin Abdelsamad, Jaouad Abari, Vedat Topsakal, Ahmet Tekin, Cila Umat, Farheen Naz Anis, Mohammad Maarefvand, Stavros Hatzopoulos, Andrea Ciorba, Piotr H. Skarzynski

First published in London, United Kingdom, 2023 by IntechOpen
IntechOpen is the global imprint of INTECHOPEN LIMITED, registered in England and Wales, registration number: 11086078, 5 Princes Gate Court, London, SW7 2QJ, United Kingdom

British Library Cataloguing-in-Publication Data
A catalogue record for this book is available from the British Library

Additional hard and PDF copies can be obtained from orders@intechopen.com

Latest Advances in Cochlear Implant Technologies and Related Clinical Applications
Edited by Stavros Hatzopoulos, Andrea Ciorba and Piotr H. Skarzynski
p. cm.
Print ISBN 978-1-83768-782-4
Online ISBN 978-1-83768-783-1
eBook (PDF) ISBN 978-1-83768-784-8

Meet the editors

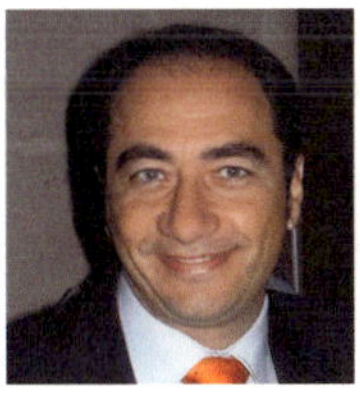

Dr. Stavros Hatzopoulos has been a faculty member of the Audiology and ENT Clinic, University of Ferrara, Italy, since 1994. His background is in biomedical engineering, audiological engineering, and hearing science. He obtained a BSc from the University of Southern California, an MSc from Texas A&M University, and a Ph.D. from Worcester Polytechnic Institute, Massachusetts, USA. He received his habilitation as an associate professor in 2014. He is the author of more than 225 book chapters, peer-reviewed papers, and congress presentations. He has participated in numerous European Concerted Action projects in otoacoustic emissions, genetics, and nanotechnologies. Dr. Hatzopoulos is the editor of the Otoacoustic Emissions Portal (www.otoemissions.org), the Audiology section editor for the *Journal of Hearing Science*, and the managing editor for *Hearing, Balance and Communication*.

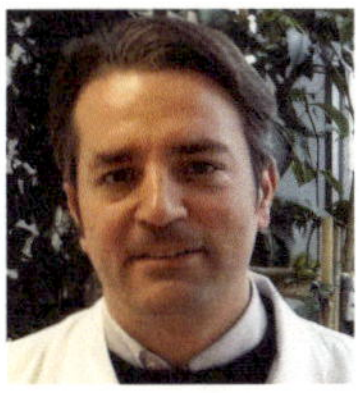

Dr. Andrea Ciorba, MD, has been a member of the Audiology and ENT Clinic, University of Ferrara, Italy, since 2004. He is the author of about 190 peer-reviewed papers and book chapters and a member of several journal editorial boards. His clinical field of interest is audiology and vestibology and he is involved in research activities in otoacoustic emissions and inner ear electrophysiology. Dr. Ciorba obtained an MD in 1999, a diploma in Otolaryngology and Head and Neck Surgery in 2003, and a Ph.D. in Audiology in 2008. He has been an Associate Professor of Audiology at the Audiology and ENT Clinic, University of Ferrara, since 2020.

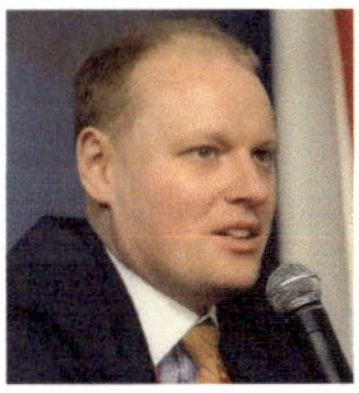

Dr. Piotr Henryk Skarzynski is a specialist in ENT, pediatric ENT, audiology and phoniatrics, and public health. He participated in the 3rd Stakeholders Consultation meeting during which the World Hearing Forum of the World Health Organization (WHO) was announced. He is a member of the WHO's Roster of Experts on Digital Health, president-elect of the International Advisory Board of the American Academy of Otolaryngology–Head and Neck Surgery (AAO-HNS), board member of the International Society for Telemedicine and eHealth (ISfTeH), and a member of the Implantable Hearing Devices Committee and Otology and Neurotology Education Committee of AAO-HNS. He is the author of more than 1156 national and international publications and 2140 conference presentations.

Contents

Preface

Latest Advances in Cochlear Implant Technologies and Related Clinical Applications reports the latest scientific and clinical research advances in cochlear implants (CIs). The volume includes chapters focusing on the anatomical challenges and surgical aspects of this hearing rehabilitation technology as well as additional areas of interest such as preoperative assessment and prosthesis fitting.

This volume was made possible through the substantial contribution of numerous authors. It is intended to complement graduate courses in audiology, speech pathology, hearing science and neurosciences, as well as basic courses in otolaryngology and audiology.

The book is organized into two sections: “CI Surgery and Related Technical Issues” and “CI Hearing Rehabilitation Strategies.”

Section I includes four chapters:

- Chapter 1: “Introductory Chapter: A Short Excursus into the Realm of Cochlear Implants Today”
- Chapter 2: “Robot-Assisted Cochlear Implant Surgery”
- Chapter 3: “Congenital Malformations of the Outer, Middle, Inner Ear and Cochlear Nerve with Favorable Cochlear Implantation”
- Chapter 4: “The Assessment of Electrode–Neuron Interface (ENI) in Cochlear Implant Users”

Section II includes five chapters:

- Chapter 5: “Anatomy-Based Programming”
- Chapter 6: “Perceptual Learning of Uncategorized Arabic Phonemes Among Congenitally Deaf, Non-native Children with Cochlear Implants”
- Chapter 7: “Perspective Chapter: Cochlear Implant Activation in the Immediate Postoperative Period at the Operating Room”
- Chapter 8: “Static Posturography with Nintendo Balance Board in Children after Cochlear Implantation”
- Chapter 9: “Auditory Neuropathy Spectrum Disorder: Genetic and Electrophysiological Testing for Predicting Rehabilitation Outcomes after Cochlear Implantation”

We would like to thank all the contributing authors and the staff at IntechOpen for their continuous and generous assistance during the preparation of this volume.

Stavros Hatzopoulos, Ph.D. and Andrea Ciorba , Ph.D.
Audiology and ENT Unit,
Department of Neurosciences and Rehabilitation,
University Hospital of Ferrara,
University of Ferrara,
Ferrara, Italy

Piotr H. Skarzynski
Institute of Sensory Organs,
Warsaw, Poland

Institute of Physiology and Pathology of Hearing,
Warsaw, Poland

Department of Heart Failure and Cardiac Rehabilitation,
Medical University of Warsaw,
Warsaw, Poland

Section 1

CI Surgery and Related Technical Issues

Chapter 1

Introductory Chapter: A Short Excursus into the Realm of Cochlear Implants Today

Andrea Ciorba, Piotr H. Skarzynski and Stavros Hatzopoulos

1. Introduction

To date, the Cochlear Implant represents a very sophisticated and effective neural prosthesis, whose hardware and software have made significant technological leaps ahead, over the last 20 years. From the two aspects of this technology, the software aspect has been particularly evolved, considering the great advancements in the area of computer science and Artificial Intelligence.

These CI prostheses are very effective in the rehabilitation of severe and profound hearing impairment cases and can be applied to the hearing rehabilitation of subjects of almost any age, from neonates to adults. In addition, data in the literature suggest that CIs can significantly enhance the perception of the quality of life, particularly in the elderly, improving self-confidence, depressive status, and eventually cognitive functions [1–5].

Future and expected advances in CI technology could involve: novel surgical approaches, introducing minimal invasive techniques for electrode insertion in order to reduce or minimize an eventual cochlear trauma; electrode reservoirs releasing locally healing and protective pharmacological agents; new stimulation protocols collecting better the residual neural responses; and an additional minimization of the hardware with optimized energy requirements and enhanced performance. It is expected that these features will significantly improve the overall stimulation of the spiral ganglion neuron population and thus will significantly improve the CI performance [1, 3, 4].

There have been reports in the literature of a CI model not requiring external hardware [3]; this could probably be quite a revolution in the clinical practice. In this case, the electrode array placed in the cochlea would be stimulated by the intact external and middle ear sound transducer and could be wirelessly recharged using a mobile phone or a special pillow charging device. However, there are still several hardware limitations, and further research is necessary before these interesting features could reach clinical use.

The most impressive impact on the CI evolution is related to the CI software development; in particular, the latest research reports findings in the area of a wider and more intelligent connectivity between the implanted device and other devices such as smartphones and smart wearables. Controlling certain aspects of the Implant via a smartphone has already reached the clinical practice. However, it is likely that in a near future, features such as remote assistance and/or a fuller remote control of the device could be further developed, offering new solutions in terms of medical follow-up in a telemedicine context [6–8].

Another important aspect of the CI development is related to the constantly increasing cost of these devices; while one could assume that hardware and software developments would be reflected in a decrease in the required implant cost, the financial reality is different. To offer the above-mentioned new technological solutions, the manufacturing companies have also increased the costs of the devices. This can generate a problem in terms of the availability of these prostheses in third-world countries.

2. Conclusion

Data in the literature suggest that the evolution of the Cochlear implant devices is constant, and many important hearing rehabilitation landmarks have already been achieved. Unfortunately, these developments are in a straight contrast with the possible diffusion of new technologies in developing third-world areas of the planet, where they are most needed.

Author details

Andrea Ciorba[1], Piotr H. Skarzynski[2,3,4] and Stavros Hatzopoulos[1*]

1 Audiology and ENT Unit, Department of Neurosciences and Rehabilitation, University Hospital of Ferrara, University of Ferrara, Ferrara, Italy

2 Institute of Sensory Organs, Warsaw, Poland

3 Institute of Physiology and Pathology of Hearing, Warsaw, Poland

4 Department of Heart Failure and Cardiac Rehabilitation, Medical University of Warsaw, Warsaw, Poland

*Address all correspondence to: sdh1@unife.it

References

[1] Ciorba A, Skarżyński PH, Gocmenler H, Hatzopoulos S. Advances in pediatric and adult Cochlear implant and middle ear prostheses. Journal of Clinical Medicine. 2021;**10**(14):3152. DOI: 10.3390/jcm10143152

[2] Aimoni C, Ciorba A, Hatzopoulos S, Ramacciotti G, Mazzoli M, Bianchini C, et al. Cochlear implants in subjects over age 65: Quality of life and Audiological outcomes. Medical Science Monitor. 2016;**22**:3035-3042. DOI: 10.12659/msm.896869

[3] Available from: https://news.mit.edu/2014/cochlear-implants-with-no-exterior-hardware-0209

[4] Wilson BS, Dorman MF. Cochlear Implants: Current designs and future possibilities. JRRD. 2008;**45**:695-730

[5] Mitchell-Innes A, Saeed S, Irving R. The future of Cochlear implant design. Advances in Oto-Rhino-Laryngology. 2018;**81**:105-113

[6] Reiss LA. Cochlear implants and other inner ear prostheses: Today and tomorrow. Current Opinion in Physiology. 2020;**18**:49-55

[7] Yao X, Liu H, Si J, Ding X, Zhao Y, Zheng Y. Research status and future development of Cochlear Reimplantation. Frontiers in Neuroscience. 2022;**16**:824389. DOI: 10.3389/fnins.2022.824389

[8] Ciorba A, Bovo R, Trevisi P, Rosignoli M, Aimoni C, Castiglione A, et al. Postoperative complications in cochlear implants: A retrospective analysis of 438 consecutive cases. European Archives of Oto-Rhino-Laryngology. 2012;**269**:1599-1603. DOI: 10.1007/s00405-011-1818-1

Chapter 2

Robot-Assisted Cochlear Implant Surgery

Jaouad Abari, Ahmet Tekin and Vedat Topsakal

Abstract

Since the inception of cochlear implantation, there has already been a lot of research into improving its technological aspects, whereas the surgical placement has enjoyed a golden standard for a long time. Since the advent of robotic surgery, there has now also been the development of robot-assisted cochlear implant surgery. This chapter will discuss the opportunities and challenges that robotic-assisted and image-guided cochlear implantation faces. The required accuracy and sensitivity to not harm inner ear structures during electrode insertion is already at the limits of human dexterity. With electrode arrays becoming smaller in the future, the need for robotic accuracy and reliability will become necessary. Robotic-assisted cochlear implantation is seen as a minimally invasive way of doing cochlear implantation surgery with the potential of being the golden standard in the future. An atraumatic intracochlear electrode array placement ensures that the anatomy and physiology of the inner ear structures are preserved as much as possible, thus reducing the risk of losing the rest of the natural hearing levels of the patient. This could lead to a broadening of the indication, opening the door for patients that only experience a loss at the higher frequencies. It is a given fact that robotising surgical procedures will standardise surgical outcomes.

Keywords: cochlear implantation, robot-assisted cochlear implant surgery (RACIS), sensorineural hearing loss (SNHL), image-guided cochlear implant surgery, autonomous middle ear access, autonomous inner ear access

1. Introduction

The implementation of robotics in cochlear implantation surgery was a step-by-step process. During the last 15 years, a lot of research went into the various components that could make robotic cochlear implant surgery a reality. Different aspects, such as designing the robot and developing safety mechanisms, were studied. It was only in 2017 that the first study was published that had combined all these different components into one functional robot [1]. Cochlear implant surgery consists of three main steps: middle ear access, inner ear access and electrode array insertion. The end goal of the implementation of robotics in cochlear implantation surgery is a fully robotic automation of these three steps. Autonomic middle ear access was the first hurdle that was overcome. Autonomic middle ear access was performed in six cases. The next hurdle of cochlear implantation surgery was autonomic inner ear access.

This hurdle was overcome in a recent study that was able to perform inner ear access in 22 out of 25 patients [2]. The last step, autonomic electrode array insertion, is a hurdle yet to be overcome. When all the hurdles are overcome, fully autonomous robotic cochlear implantation surgery will become a reality.

A key question being asked is why we should aim for a full robotic automation of cochlear implantation surgery. Conventional cochlear implantation surgery is already well established, in which the risk of complications is minimised under an experienced surgeon. The facial recess approach, widely seen as the golden standard, has consistently achieved a facial nerve injury rate of less than 1% [3]. Still, with conventional cochlear implantation surgery, an atraumatic electrode array insertion into the scala tympani of the cochlea cannot be ensured. Stereocilia in the cochlea are very susceptible to damage. Robotic cochlear implantation surgery could predict and minimise the trauma during electrode array insertion thus preserving the residual hearing of the patient, widening the indication of surgery. Robotic cochlear implantation surgery would also have a great impact on healthcare costs and the time under general anaesthesia. The conventional method of cochlear implantation surgery can be within 1 hour within the hands of an experienced surgeon. Robotic cochlear implantation surgery would take less than 10 minutes for inner ear access without the safety protocols that are currently in place. With the further development of robotic cochlear implantation surgery, it would potentially become an outpatient procedure under local anaesthesia.

2. Robot-assisted cochlear implant surgery

Robot-assisted cochlear implant surgery (RACIS) would not have been able to develop without the advances made in image-guidance technology. In 2014, a study was published that sought to reach the round window in a minimally invasive way [4]. The ideal insertion into the inner ear is defined as an insertion through the round window with the trajectory being parallel to the basal turn of the cochlea as long as possible, in order to not hurt any inner ear structures. If one would like to follow this definition of the most efficient path to the round window, one would have to drill through the facial nerve. The ideal drilling trajectory is by definition deviating from the optimal trajectory. Clinical research though has to show that perhaps another definition is better because, inevitably, every trajectory is bound to hit the lateral wall of the inner ear. It may be shown that trajectories that are hitting the lateral wall more basal could have perhaps a better preservation of the apical structures. Currently, these data are not available.

This shows the importance of preoperative imaging. Using preoperative imaging, an attempt was made to create a trajectory to the round window where there is a safe distance between the drill and critical structures. The aim was an insertion through the round window with the trajectory being parallel to the basal turn of the cochlea as long as possible. This would, therefore, allow electrode insertion to be easier and less traumatic. Labadie et al. reported a study with nine patients where they had managed to implant eight patients [4]. In six of these patients, the electrode arrays were completely in the scala tympani of the cochlea. The electrode arrays were placed through a cochleostomy after lifting a tympanomeatal flap. During the study, there were some complications such as the tip folding-over and facial nerve injury because of the heat created during drilling. In one patient, a switch to the conventional method was necessary because of difficulties met during electrode array insertion. A frame was used during drilling. This way, deviations of the trajectory could be led to a minimum.

Intraoperatively, two CT scans were taken for verifying if the intraoperative trajectory was not deviating from the planned trajectory. A second safety mechanism used during drilling was the use of intraoperative facial nerve monitoring, which is also used in the conventional method of cochlear implantation. Post-operatively, a final CT scan followed to verify if the electrode array was positioned correctly.

In 2017, the first system, termed the OtoBot system and surgical workflow for robot-assisted cochlear implant surgery, was developed [5]. The workflow is described as follows. After the indication for cochlear implantation is made, a screening CT is done. In current safety protocols, a risk mitigation of facial nerve palsy is defined as the distance between the planned trajectory and the course of the facial nerve being three standard deviations larger than the accuracy of the system Caversaccio et al. reported the first study in men using the OtoBot system for robotic middle ear access for cochlear implantation. A total of nine patients were included in the study. The procedure had to be converted to conventional surgery in three out of the nine patients because of safety reasons. In one of the six patients where middle ear access was performed, the insertion of the electrode array in the scala tympani was not possible because of a plaque formation in the cochlear basal turn in a patient with Cogan syndrome. A complete insertion of the electrode array in the scala tympani of the cochlea was reported in two out of the six patients [6].

The patient's anatomy has to be screened for suitability for the robot to drill a safe trajectory. Using OTOPLAN®, a dedicated planning software, a 3D reconstruction of the images and a simulation of the trajectory are made. After the anaesthesia and immobilisation of the patient, several fiducial screws are placed with imaging again after this. A simulation of the trajectory is again made after this. Once the trajectory is confirmed, robotic drilling starts in several steps. Between these different steps, imaging and facial nerve monitoring are used to check whether one is on the right trajectory. The drilling ends when an access to the middle ear is made.

2.1 Preoperative imaging and planning

A screening CT will confirm whether the patient's anatomy allows a safe route to the round window. Using a software programme, such as OTOPLAN®, a 3D reconstruction of the anatomy is made. All the anatomical parameters, such as the size of the facial recess, cochlear length and angles of cochlear approach, are segmented. The facial recess is the distance between the facial nerve and the chorda tympani. Using OTOPLAN®, a simulation of the trajectory is made (see **Figure 1**). The average size of the facial recess is 2.54 ± 0.5 mm. In this space, a drill of 1.8-mm diameter has to pass at a safe distance from both the facial nerve and the chorda tympani [7]. Currently, for the risk mitigation of facial nerve palsy, a minimum distance of 0.4 mm from the facial nerve is used. This distance is defined as the distance between the planned trajectory and the course of the facial nerve being three standard deviations larger than the accuracy of the system. Ansó et al. reported that facial nerve monitoring was able to prevent the structural damage of the facial nerve at this distance with great sensitivity and specificity [7]. They have shown that a customised facial nerve monitoring device using both the active mono- and bipolar stimulations was able to guide drilling through the facial recess safely in an animal model trial. Ansó et al. also assessed the performance of the customised facial nerve monitoring device in smaller distances between 0.1 and 0.4 mm in animal experiments [8]. The study concluded that between these respective distances, facial nerve monitoring was also able to avoid structural damage. All the trajectories with distances greater than 0.1 mm were

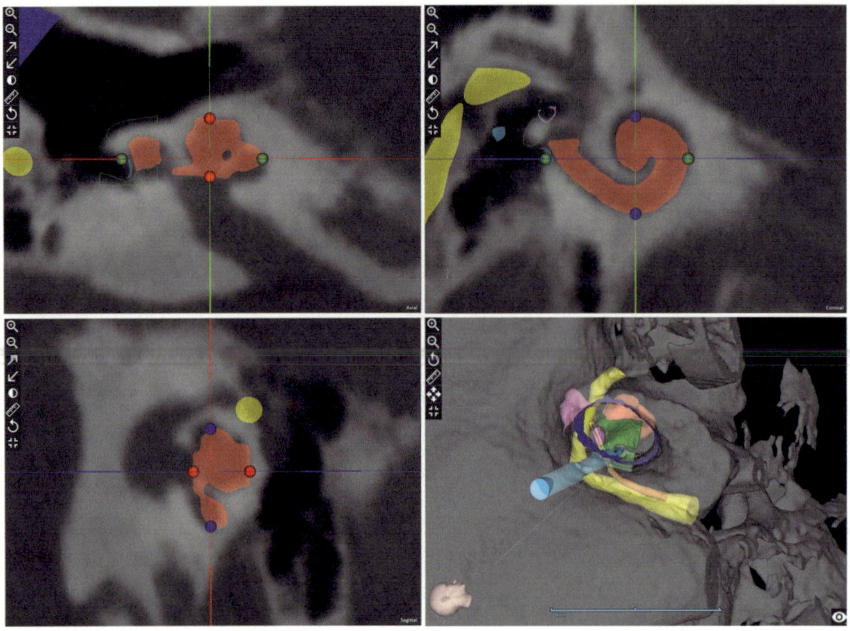

Figure 1.
A simulation of the optimal robotic drilling trajectory using planning software (OTOPLAN).

correctly classified as being uncritical to continue drilling. In distances closer than 0.1 mm, however, facial nerve monitoring was able to assess a correct distance in only four out of the seven trajectories. This study only assessed for structural facial nerve damage and did not investigate the post-operative functional status.

RACIS starts with placing the head of the patient in an atraumatic head rest. Pinning the patient's skull as in certain neurosurgical procedures is, therefore, not necessary. After a conventional retro-auricular incision, the placement of about four fiducial screws on the surface of the mastoid follows. These will serve as artificial landmarks on imaging and are important for the registration of the images. One additional fiducial is placed to hold a patient marker. Registration comprises the robot with a fused image of both the preoperative images and the working surface in which the surgeon has to operate. This is visualised with a camera. It also verifies if the planned trajectory meets the safety settings towards critical structures. After a safe trajectory is reconfirmed on OTOPLAN®, the operation can follow.

2.2 Autonomous middle ear access

The surgical robot currently used RACIS is the HEARO® robotic system developed by CASCINATION in Switzerland (see **Figure 2**). The accuracy and precision was described as 0.1 ± 0.05 mm when verified with a laser scanner and 0.15 ± 0.08 mm when verified on human cadavers [1].

The very first step of autonomous middle ear approach is the robotic drilling from the surface of the mastoid to around 3 mm in front of the estimated depth of the facial nerve. This step is done in 2-mm intervals where it is important to properly clean the drilled cavity between each step with saline water. The importance of flushing and working in intervals is necessary to avoid excess heat during drilling. Drilling is stopped 3 mm in front of the estimated depth of the facial nerve, and the first

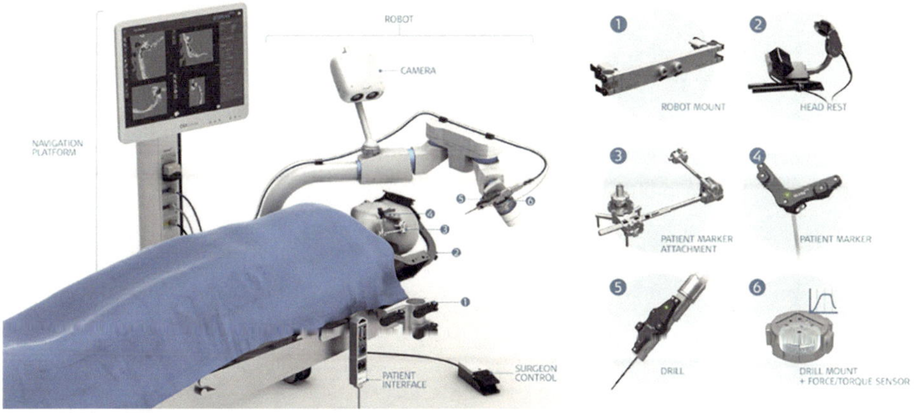

Figure 2.
The HEARO® robotic system. (1) robot mount, (2) headrest, (3) patient marker attachment, (4) patient marker, (5) drill and (6) drill mount with force/torque sensor [2].

intraoperative CT is performed to evaluate the distance of the drilled trajectory but also to calculate any inaccuracies. Here, it is important that a titanium rod is placed inside the drilled cavity. This will ensure that one will be able to differentiate the drilled trajectory from the surrounding anatomy more easily. The drilled trajectory is compared with the planned trajectory during this step, and the decision to continue drilling or not is made. Intraoperative imaging is done with a mobile cone-beam CT that has a spatial resolution of at least 0.1 mm.

The second step of autonomous middle ear approach is the most critical step, drilling in the facial recess between the facial nerve and the chorda tympani. This involves drilling in 0.5-mm intervals until just beyond the facial nerve. It is crucial to maintain a minimum distance of 0.4 mm from the facial nerve and 0.3 mm from the chorda tympani during this step. Between each interval, it is necessary to confirm the safety of the drilled trajectory with neuromonitoring what will be repeated five times in the course of the second step [4].

The third step of the operation is the fastest and least critical step. Drilling will continue until one reaches the middle ear. In this step, there is the least risk of damaging critical structures (see **Figure 3**).

2.3 Autonomous inner ear access

Autonomous inner ear access is the next step after autonomous middle ear access and is performed with a 1.0-mm burr instead of a 1.8-mm drill. Topsakal et al. reported successful minimally invasive autonomous inner ear access in 22 out of 25 patients [2]. All the 22 cases were performed safely with no reports of complications. RACIS was aborted in three out of the 25 cases during autonomous middle ear access, after the first intraoperative CT was taken. These three cases were converted to conventional cochlear implantation surgery because either a sufficient intraoperative accuracy could not be guaranteed due to software failure (two cases) or the evaluation of the trajectory was not determined to be safe (one case).

The process of autonomous inner ear access is the milling of the bony overhang of the round window, also referred to as the canonus fossulae fenestrae cochlea or canonus in short [9]. It covers the round window for a part and serves as a protection

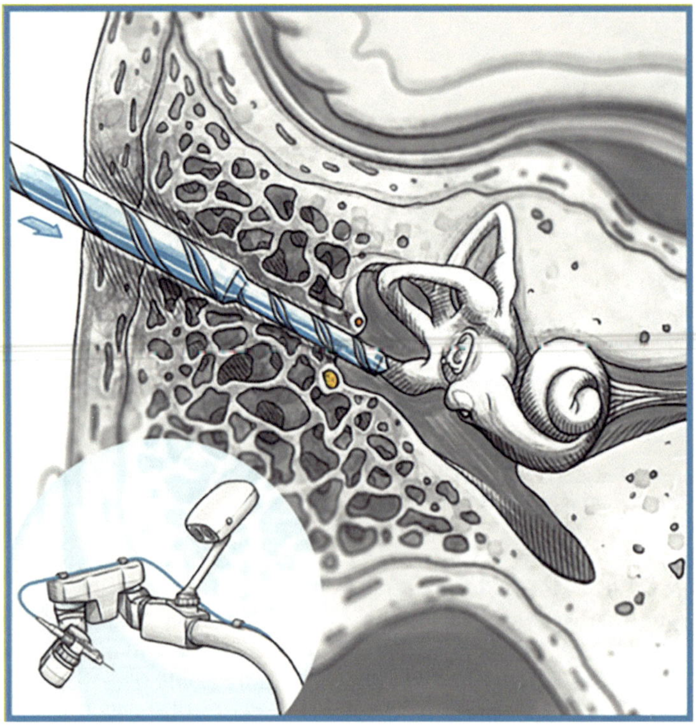

Figure 3.
The HEARO®-robotic system drilling through the mastoid with a 1.8-mm drill performing middle ear access. Facial nerve (yellow) and Chorda tympani (red) [2].

of the round window. This access is required to be able to pass a 0.8-mm-diameter electrode array through the 1-mm-diameter canonostomy (see **Figure 4**), whereas in conventional surgery, a full canonectomy needs to be performed to have visual confirmation of the round window and, if possible, the course of the basal turn. A minimal invasive inner ear access and electrode insertion can be ensured with this procedure being image guided. The thickness of the canonus is calculated using preoperative imaging. Both its lateral and medial limits are also defined. The position of the mill during the milling process can always be calculated intraoperatively by using a force-torque sensor that is connected to the robotic arm that is performing the milling process.

The process of autonomous inner access is divided into four phases (see **Figures 5** and **6**). Phase 1 or the touchdown phase is when the drill comes into contact with the lateral wall of the canonus. Here, the force-torque sensor will measure a sudden increase in force because of a sudden increase in resistance. Phase 2 or the plateau phase is when the drill is fully positioned inside the canonus. Here, the resistance remains the same, and the force-torque sensor will always measure the same force. Phase 3 or the breakthrough phase starts when the drill has reached the medial wall of the canonus. Because of a decrease in the thickness of the bone, there will also be a decrease in the resistance that has to be overcome by the drill bit. This is also illustrated by a decrease in force. In phase 4 or the enlarging phase, the drill must still drill 0.3 mm beyond the edge of the medial wall. As a result, the diameter of the canonostomy will be equal to 1.0 mm throughout its trajectory, and the electrode array with a diameter of 0.8 mm will be able to be inserted smoothly.

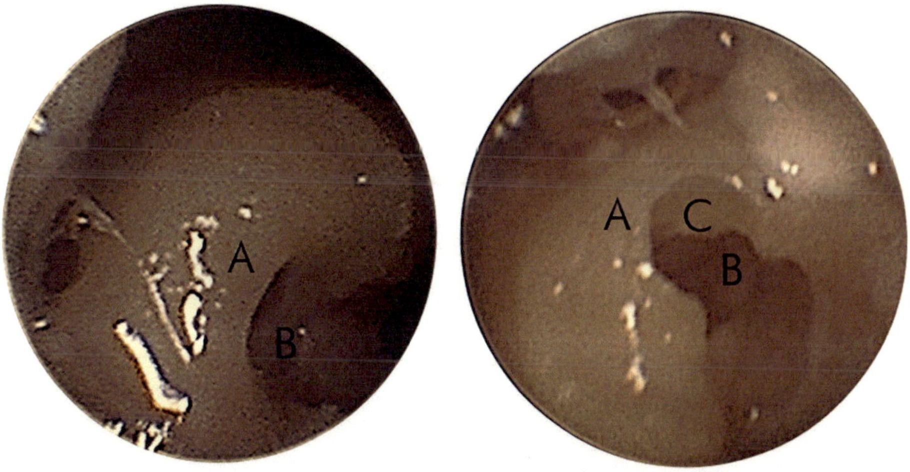

Figure 4.
An endoscopic view of the canonus (A), the round window (B) and a partial canonectomy (C) [2].

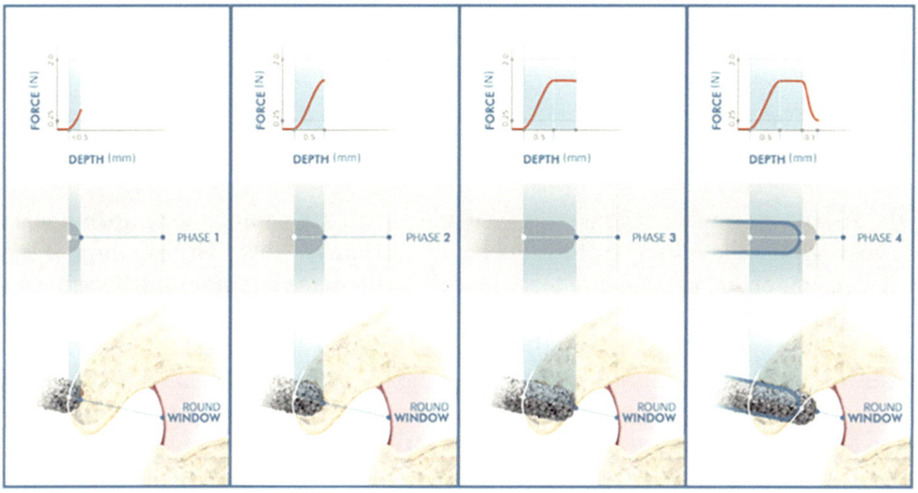

Figure 5.
Inner ear access algorithm [2].

2.4 Last step: Autonomous electrode placement

Although there are currently already some telemanipulators that can assist the insertion of an electrode array at a certain pace in standardised feed rates, such as the RobOtol® system [10] and the iotaSOFT® system [11], none of these warrants a standardised insertion angle towards the inner ear.

In this definition, an autonomous electrode placement has not yet been realised in clinical practice. In the HEARO procedure, this step is still done manually by the surgeon (see **Figure 6**). Because of the minimal invasiveness of RACIS, visualising the electrode array during insertion in the drilled trajectory is not possible. To make insertion possible, the surgeon will try to visualise the round window via the external auditory canal and by folding over the tympanic membrane. This way, a visualisation

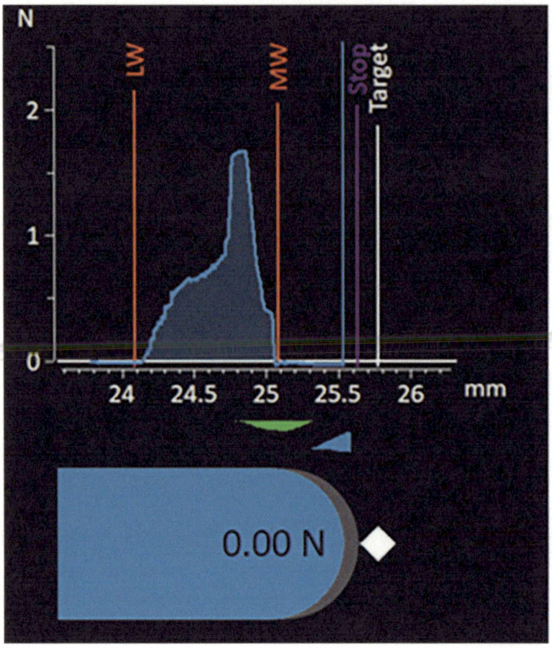

Figure 6.
Intraoperative use of the inner ear access algorithm describing the force and the depth during canonostomy; the lateral wall (LW) and the medial wall (MW).

of the electrode array during insertion is made possible. Opening the tympanomeatal flap goes against the principle of RACIS being a minimally invasive procedure. It is, therefore, important to develop a technique that allows the autonomous placement of the electrode array. After a series of 30 cases, Topsakal et al. managed to fine-tune the insertion angles and round window approach to develop in 2022 a new clinical routine for inserting electrodes without opening the tympanomeatal flap. The design of a device that is capable of inserting the electrode at an automated speed would not be too difficult. Calibrating and defining the insertion angles before the approval of a surgeon would expect a learning curve.

Topsakal et al. reported a successful and complete insertion of the electrode array in 21 out of the 22 cases. Twenty-five patients were included in the study, but three had to be converted to conventional surgery because of safety protocols. In one case out of the 22 cases, the angle of insertion proved to be problematic with the last contact of the electrode (C12) being localised in the position of the round window [2]. In three out of the 22 cases, electrode array insertion was not possible from the first time. Because of a difficult angle of insertion in two cases, it was decided to enlarge the round window approach. In one case, an intracochlear ossification in a patient with Cogan syndrome hindered a smooth insertion. Here, it was decided to widen the inner ear space. A successful electrode insertion was eventually possible in all the three patients. During electrode array insertion, a guiding tube is used to avoid a false route to aerated mastoid cells (**Figure 7**). The guiding tube exits out of two half pieces allowing for an easy removal after electrode array insertion. The guiding tube still allows the surgeon to estimate the depth of electrode insertion. All the electrode array insertions in this study were done with a 28-mm straight flexible lateral wall electrode (Med-EL, Innsbruck, Austria). The guiding tubes allow for a quick and easy electrode

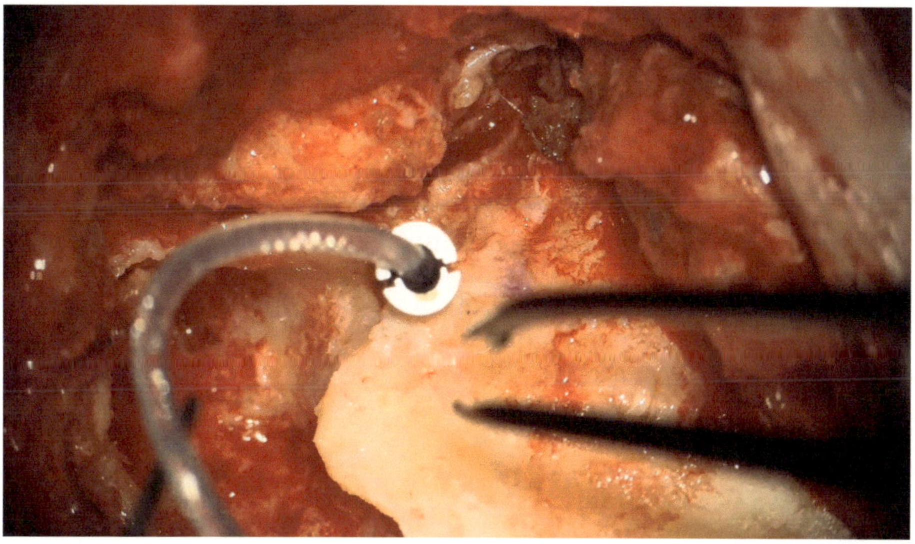

Figure 7.
Manual insertion of the electrode array using a guiding tube.

insertion with these flexible electrode arrays. Post-operatively, a final cone-beam CT follows. A correct position of the electrode is checked this way. Electrophysiological tests are also used to check if the electrode array is fully inserted.

Rajan et al. reported in a study of 40 patients that a slower speed of electrode array insertion leads to a better preservation of the patient's residual hearing and vestibular function [12]. Here, two speeds of insertion were compared, namely, a speed of 15 and 60 mm/min. The mean loss at low frequencies in dB was 16 ± 1.75 in the high-speed insertion group and 10.5 ± 2.5 in the low-speed insertion group. This conclusion was carried over to the development of the autonomous systems.

In ref. [13], different types of motoric insertion of electrode arrays were studied in *in vitro* models of the scala tympani. Here, more than 1000 insertions were studied. It was concluded that the smoothness of the insertion could be greatly improved, and the necessary forces could be greatly reduced depending on the angle at which the electrode array was inserted. This angle is the angle relative to the centre line of the scala tympani. The smoothest insertion corresponds with the electrode array running parallel to this centreline. In this study, it was also shown that a non-constant speed of electrode insertion also leads to a decrease in the amount of force required to do the insertion. The speed of insertion should decrease depending on the progression of electrode array insertion. Less force would mean that the insertion would be less traumatic.

The technical knowledge of the most optimal electrode insertion will be used to make RACIS a fully automated process from middle ear access to electrode insertion. This knowledge will help standardise results in terms of residual hearing after the procedure.

3. Conclusion

RACIS has demonstrated to be safe and reliable for cochlear implantation. It has the potential to standardise the surgical outcomes of cochlear implantation to a maximum. When mechanical trauma is also limited to the bare minimum, it may pave the way for new indications for cochlear implantation in terms of electroacoustic simulation. The thrive to improve RACIS has already contributed a lot to the healthcare of patients with sensorineural hearing loss. The tools in image guidance surgery have shown us the importance of an individualised patient care because of the differences in cochlear duct length [14].

As a minimal invasive technique, RACIS requires only a canonostomy, whereas in conventional surgery, a full canonectomy needs to be performed to have visual confirmation of the round window and, if possible, the course of the basal turn.

Every trajectory to the inner ear is bound to hit the lateral wall of the inner ear. It may be shown that trajectories that are hitting the lateral wall more basal could have perhaps a better preservation of the apical structures. Currently, these data are not available.

The indication for RACIS versus conventional surgery is still strict. Currently, with the use of a drill of 1.8 mm, it is estimated that 50–75% of patients are indicated to be operated on via the RACIS technique. With future developments and the drill getting smaller to 1.0 mm, it is expected that RACIS would be possible in up to 100% of the patients [15]. The HEARO procedure is still not a fully autonomous way of cochlear implantation surgery, with autonomous electrode array insertion being not yet clinically possible. Further studies into making the procedure more efficient and safe are to be expected.

Acknowledgements

Prof. Vedat Topsakal enjoys a senior research grant from FWO Vlaanderen number 18B3222N.

All authors would like to thank MED-EL (Innsbruck, Austria) and CAScination (Bern, Switzerland) for their support for this project.

Conflict of interest

The authors declare no conflict of interest.

Author details

Jaouad Abari*, Ahmet Tekin and Vedat Topsakal
Department of Otorhinolaryngology Head and Neck Surgery, University Hospital UZ Brussel, Vrije Universiteit Brussel, Brussels, Belgium

*Address all correspondence to: abdeljaouad.abari@uzbrussel.be

References

[1] Weber S, Gavaghan K, Wimmer W, Williamson T, Gerber N, Anso J, et al. Instrument flight to the inner ear. Science Robotics. 2017;**2**(4):eaa14916. DOI: 10.1126/scirobotics.aal4916

[2] Topsakal V, Heuninck E, Matulic M, Tekin AM, Mertens G, Van Rompaey V, et al. First study in men evaluating a surgical robotic tool providing autonomous inner ear access for cochlear implantation. Frontiers in Neurology. 2022;**2022**:13. DOI: 10.3389/fneur.2022.804507

[3] Thom JJ, Carlson ML, Olson MD, Neff BA, Beatty CW, Facer GW, et al. The prevalence and clinical course of facial nerve paresis following cochlear implant surgery. The Laryngoscope. 2013;**132**(4):1000-1004. DOI: 10.1002/lary.23316

[4] Labadie RF, Balachandran R, Noble JH, Blachon GS, Mitchell JE, Reda FA, et al. Minimally invasive image-guided cochlear implantation surgery: First report of clinical implementation. The Laryngoscope. 2014;**124**(8):1915-1922. DOI: 10.1002/lary.24520

[5] Caversaccio M, Gavaghan K, Wimmer W, Williamson T, Ansò J, Mantokoudis G, et al. Robotic cochlear implantation: Surgical procedure and first clinical experience. Acta Oto-Laryngologica. 2017;**137**(4):447-454. DOI: 10.1080/00016489.2017.1278573

[6] Caversaccio M, Wimmer W, Anso J, Mantokoudis G, Gerber N, Rathgeb C, et al. Robotic middle ear access for cochlear implantation: First in man. PLoS One. 2019;**14**(8):Article e0220543. DOI: 10.1371/journal.pone.0220543

[7] Ansó J, Scheidegger O, Wimmer W, Gavaghan K, Gerber N, Schneider D, et al. Neuromonitoring during robotic Cochlear implantation: Initial clinical experience. Annals of Biomedical Engineering. 2018;**46**(10):1568-1581. DOI: 10.1007/s10439-018-2094-7

[8] Ansó J, Dür C, Apelt M, Venail F, Scheidegger O, Seidel K, et al. Prospective validation of facial nerve monitoring to prevent nerve damage during robotic drilling. Frontiers in Surgery. 2019;**2019**:6. DOI: 10.3389/fsurg.2019.00058

[9] Topsakal V, Kachlik D, Bahşi I, Carlson M, Isaacson B, Broman J, et al. Relevant temporal bone anatomy for robotic cochlear implantation: An updated terminology combined with anatomical and clinical terms. Translational Research in Anatomy. 2021;**25**:100138. DOI: 10.1016/j.tria.2021.100138

[10] Vittoria S, Lahlou G, Torres R, Daoudi H, Mosnier I, Mazalaigue S, et al. Robot-based assistance in middle ear surgery and cochlear implantation: First clinical report. European Archives of Oto-Rhino-Laryngology. 2020;**2020**:26. DOI: 10.1007/s00405-020-06070-z

[11] Kaufmann CR, Henslee AM, Claussen A, Hansen MR. Evaluation of insertion forces and cochlea trauma following robotics-assisted cochlear implant electrode array insertion. Otology & Neurotology. 2022;**41**(5):631-638. DOI: 10.1097/mao.0000000000002608

[12] Rajan GP, Kontorinis G, Kuthubutheen J. The effects of insertion speed on inner ear function during Cochlear implantation: A comparison study. Audiology and Neurotology. 2013;**18**(1):17-22. DOI: 10.1159/000342821

[13] Aebischer P, Mantokoudis G, Weder S, Anschuetz L, Caversaccio M, Wimmer W. In-vitro study of speed and alignment angle in cochlear implant electrode array insertions. IEEE Transactions on Biomedical Engineering. 2021;**2021**:1. DOI: 10.1109/tbme.2021.3088232

[14] Mertens G, Van Rompaey V, Van de Heyning P, Gorris E, Topsakal V. Prediction of the cochlear implant electrode insertion depth: Clinical applicability of two analytical cochlear models. Scientific Reports. 2020;**10**(1):24. DOI: 10.1038/s41598-020-58648-6

[15] Auinger AB, Dahm V, Liepins R, Riss D, Baumgartner WD, Arnoldner C. Robotic cochlear implant surgery: Imaging-based evaluation of feasibility in clinical routine. Frontiers in Surgery. 2021;**8**:29. DOI: 10.3389/fsurg.2021.742219

Chapter 3

Congenital Malformations of the Outer, Middle, Inner Ear and Cochlear Nerve with Favorable Cochlear Implantation

Liia V. Toropchina and Elena I. Zelikovich

Abstract

This case study presents the neuroradiological findings of two deaf children with CHARGE syndrome and oculo-auriculo-vertebral spectrum disease. Both patients had rare combinations of ear and auditory nerve anomalies associated with a high risk of intra- and postoperative complications during cochlear implantation (CI) and poor results. However, CI was carried out with favorable results in terms of hearing and speech development. When determining indications for CI in children with complex anomalies, it is necessary to assess the state of all ear structures in computed tomography of the temporal bones and MR (3 Tesla) images. The most critical is the state of the following structures: cochlea—modiolus—cochlear aperture—diameter of the internal auditory canal—the presence and condition of the auditory nerve. In the presence of a normal or dysplastic cochlea, a hypoplastic auditory nerve is not a contraindication for CI. In this situation, the presence of a modiolus and at least partially open cochlear aperture are prognostically favorable. In the presence of a large or small common cavity, an undivided vestibulocochlear nerve is not considered a contraindication for CI. Such a combination—a common cavity and an undivided vestibulocochlear nerve—is a prognostically quite favorable option.

Keywords: temporal bone anomalies, congenital malformations of the inner ear, common cavity, stenosis/bone obliteration of the cochlear aperture, stenosis of the internal auditory canal, anomalies of the facial nerve canal, hypoplasia/aplasia of the cochlear nerve, cochlear implantation, CHARGE syndrome, oculo-auriculo- vertebral spectrum, OAVS, CT of the temporal bones, MRI 3T of the cochlear nerves

1. Introduction

Congenital malformations of the inner ear structures can occur in various combinations and be combined with anomalies of the outer and middle ear, as well as aplasia/hypoplasia of the cochlear nerve. At the same time, aplasia/hypoplasia of the cochlear nerve can occur both in stenotic and normal internal auditory canal (IAC).

Regarding the anomalies of the inner ear, the greatest doubts in terms of the prospects of cochlear implantation (CI) are the absence or induration of the modiolus, stenosis/obliteration of the cochlear aperture and the dubious condition of the cochlear nerve [1].

Abnormal middle ear anatomy affects surgical landmarks and in some cases makes it difficult to identify the cochlea [2]. The absence of the auditory nerve is a contraindication to surgery, and the correct assessment of its condition in case of hypoplasia essentially determines the fate of a deaf child.

CI in cases of severe combined ear anomalies is associated with a high risk of intra and postoperative complications and poor results. To determine the indications for cochlear implantation in children with complex temporal bone malformations, it is necessary to perform high-resolution computed tomography (CT) of the temporal bones and 3 T magnetic resonance imaging (MRI) of the cochlear nerves. The results of the studies should be evaluated by an experienced radiologist to determine contraindications and assess the likelihood of intraoperative complications. The increase in the number of such patients requires clear indications for CI, as it has an economic interest.

There is an opinion that modern imaging methods cannot accurately reflect the state of the cochlear nerve or predict the benefit of CI for a child [3]. The presence of several anomalies of the temporal bone further complicates the decision to operate. Therefore, the demonstration of variants of complex combined anomalies with a positive effect of CI is useful for resolving the issue of surgery when faced with similar cases.

Particularly complex combined malformations of the temporal bone structures occur in CHARGE syndrome (CS) [4] and in diseases of the oculo-auriculo-vertebral spectrum (OAVS) [5].

2. Objective

To report the neuroradiological findings of two deaf children with CS and OAVS who underwent CI with favorable outcomes in terms of hearing and language development.

3. Materials and methods

Two children (male and female), one with CS, the other with OAVS, who, according to a comprehensive audiological examination (OAE, impedance, auditory evoked potentials and hearing aid fitting) had bilateral total deafness.

High-resolution CT was performed on a GE Revolution Discovery CT tomograph.

MRI of the brain with a targeted study of the cochlear nerves and intravenous contrast enhancement with a gadovist was performed on a GE 3 T Discovery 750 tomograph according to the technique described by Glastonbury C. M. et al. [6].

4. Results

Case 1. Young female I., born in 2017, with phenotypic signs of CS. There was a delay in physical development. She was observed by an ophthalmologist with diagnoses—coloboma of the optic nerve and choroid, microcornea, microphthalmos, complex astigmatism and non-permanent concomitant convergent strabismus. The child has auricular dysplasia, more on the right, audiological screening failed in both ears. A comprehensive audiological examination at the age of 4 months established a bilateral severe hearing loss. The young female was fitted with powerful hearing aids and spoke short, simple words (mom, dad). In the first 3 years of life, gradually progressive hearing loss was noted, with some fluctuation of hearing thresholds, from severe hearing loss to complete deafness. The super-power hearing aids had no effect.

CT of the temporal bones revealed a bilateral congenital anomaly of the middle and inner ear. On both sides, the anvil-malleolar complex and the long process of the incus were formed correctly. The stirrup is large, and fixation of the posterior leg to the canal of the facial nerve is noted. The oval window is reduced, compacted, and the round window is formed correctly. The vestibule is somewhat expanded. The cochlear aqueducts are formed correctly. The vestibule aqueduct is narrow. The semicircular canals are not formed. The IAC has a diameter of 4 mm. The facial nerve canal is formed typically, and the bone walls are preserved. Lateralization of the sigmoid sinus is noted.

On the right, the cochlea is dysplastically formed, and the apical turn is somewhat reduced. The modiolus and its base are considerably compacted. The aperture of the cochlea is sharply narrowed and compacted (**Figure 1a–d**).On the left, the cochlea is formed with incomplete separation of the curls. The number of turns has been reduced. The modiolus is not visible. The area of the cochlear aperture is completely covered by bone tissue (**Figure 2a–d**).

Conclusion—CT picture of bilateral anomaly of the stapes, fenestra vestibule, aplasia of the semicircular canals, cochlear dysplasia, stenosis and partial obliteration of the cochlear aperture on the right and complete obliteration of the cochlear aperture on the left.

MRI 3 T—On the right—hypoplasia of the cochlear nerve (filiform) (**Figure 1e**), on the left—aplasia of the cochlear nerve (**Figure 2e**). The council decided to perform CI on the right ear. After the operation, she regularly works with a speech and language pathologist, understands addressed speech and speaks in phrases.

Case 2. Young male T., born in 2021. At birth, OAVS was established, a normal male karyotype. DiGeorge syndrome and velocardiofacial syndrome have been ruled out by genetic tests, and genome sequencing is underway. The child has a transverse cleft of the face, bilateral microtia, narrow external auditory canals and appendages of the auricles. A comprehensive audiological examination revealed bilateral complete deafness. Attempts of the super-power hearing aids fitting of air and bone conduction were ineffective.

CT of the temporal bones—on both sides—the mastoid process has a cellular system, developed according to age, the pneumatization of which is not disturbed. The external auditory canal has a diameter of 6 mm. The bone part of the auditory tube and the tympanic cavity are pneumatized. The facial nerve canal can be traced only in the mastoid part. The canal of the internal carotid artery is not clearly visible. The fossa of the jugular vein and the sigmoid sinus is determined.

On the right, the auditory ossicles are represented by the malleus, anvil and arch of the stirrup. The footplate of the stirrup is not formed. The medial wall of the tympanic cavity is formed abnormally. The structures of the inner ear are represented by a single large cystic cavity, a fragment of which, 3x5 mm in size, prolapses like a hernia into the tympanic cavity through a 2 mm hole in the medial wall. IAC has a diameter of 0.5 mm (**Figure 3a–f**).

On the left, the auditory ossicles are represented by the malleus, an incus with a dysplastic long process and an arch of the stirrup. The footplate of the stirrup is not

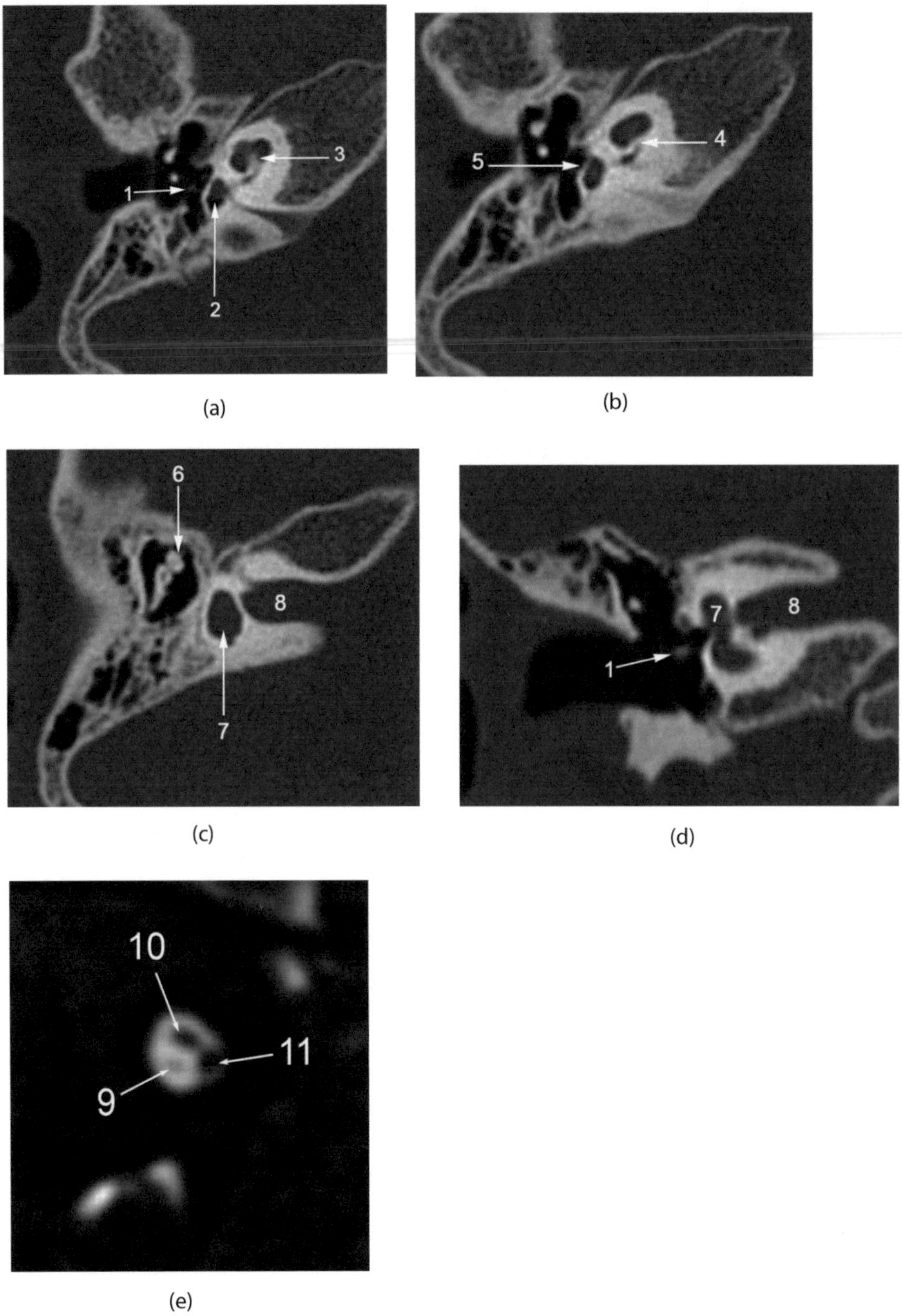

Figure 1.
(a–e) Young female I., CS. Axial and coronary tomograms of the right temporal bone. 1—large stirrup, 2—well-formed round window, 3—the modiolus is significantly compacted, 4—the cochlear aperture is sharply narrowed, compacted, 5—the oval window is reduced in size, compacted, 6—the anvil-hammer complex is not changed, 7—the vestibule is somewhat expanded, the semicircular canals are absent, 8—the internal auditory canal has a normal diameter, 9—cochlear nerve, 10—facial nerve and 11—vestibular nerve.

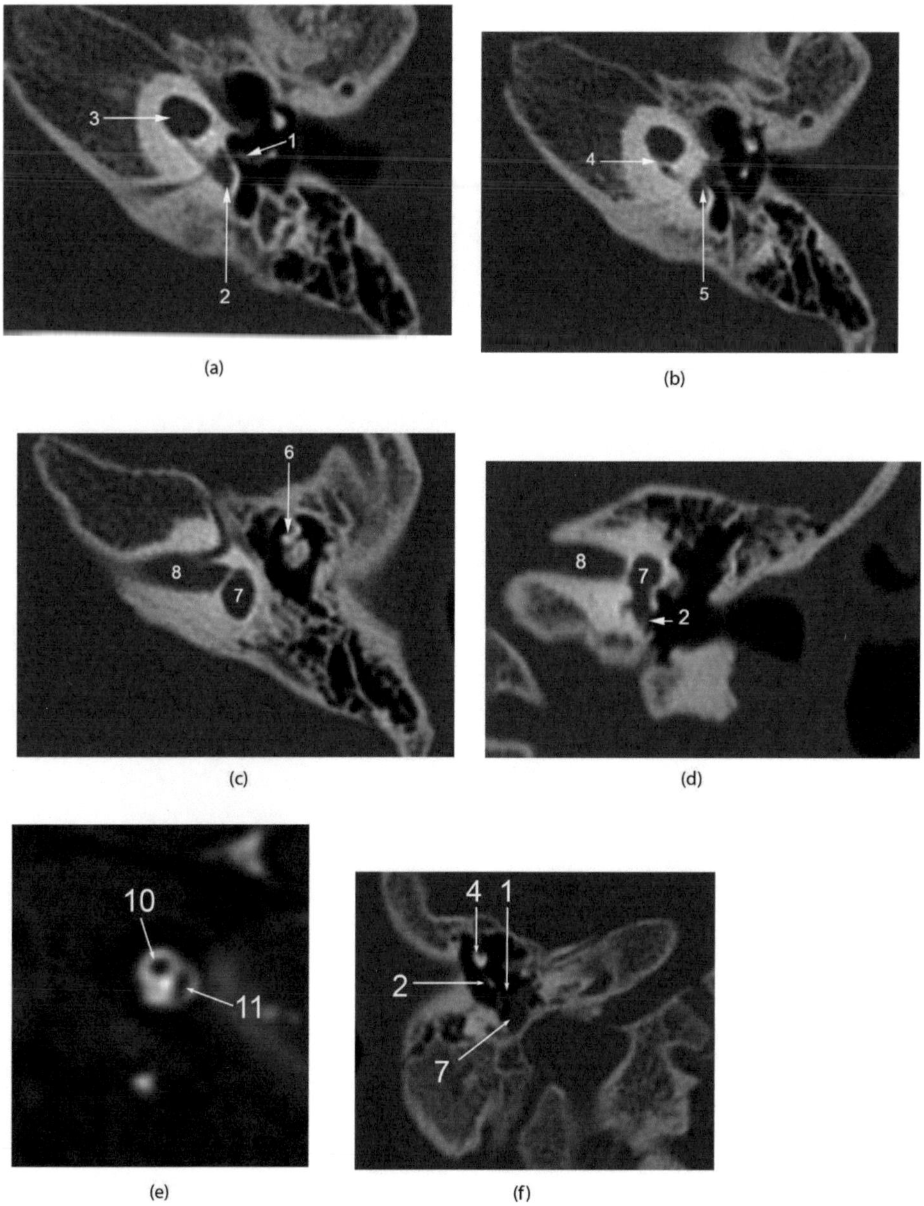

Figure 2.
(a–e) Young female I., CS. Axial and coronary tomograms of the left temporal bone. 1—large stirrup, 2—correctly formed round window, 3—incomplete separation of the cochlear turns with a decrease in their size, the modiolus is absent, 4—the cochlear aperture is closed by bone tissue, 5—the oval window is reduced in size, compacted, 6—the anvil-malleolar complex is not changed, 7—the vestibule is somewhat expanded, the semicircular canals are absent, 8—the internal auditory canal has a normal diameter, 10—facial nerve and 11—vestibular nerve.

formed. The medial wall of the tympanic cavity is formed abnormally. The structures of the inner ear are represented by a single cystic cavity of small size. IAC has a diameter of 1 mm (**Figure 4a–f**).

Conclusion—CT picture of a bilateral congenital anomaly of the middle and inner ear. On the right—a large common cavity prolapses like a hernia into the tympanic cavity. Severe stenosis of the IAC. Anomaly of the facial nerve canal. On the left is a small common cavity. Stenosis of the IAC. Anomaly of the facial nerve canal.

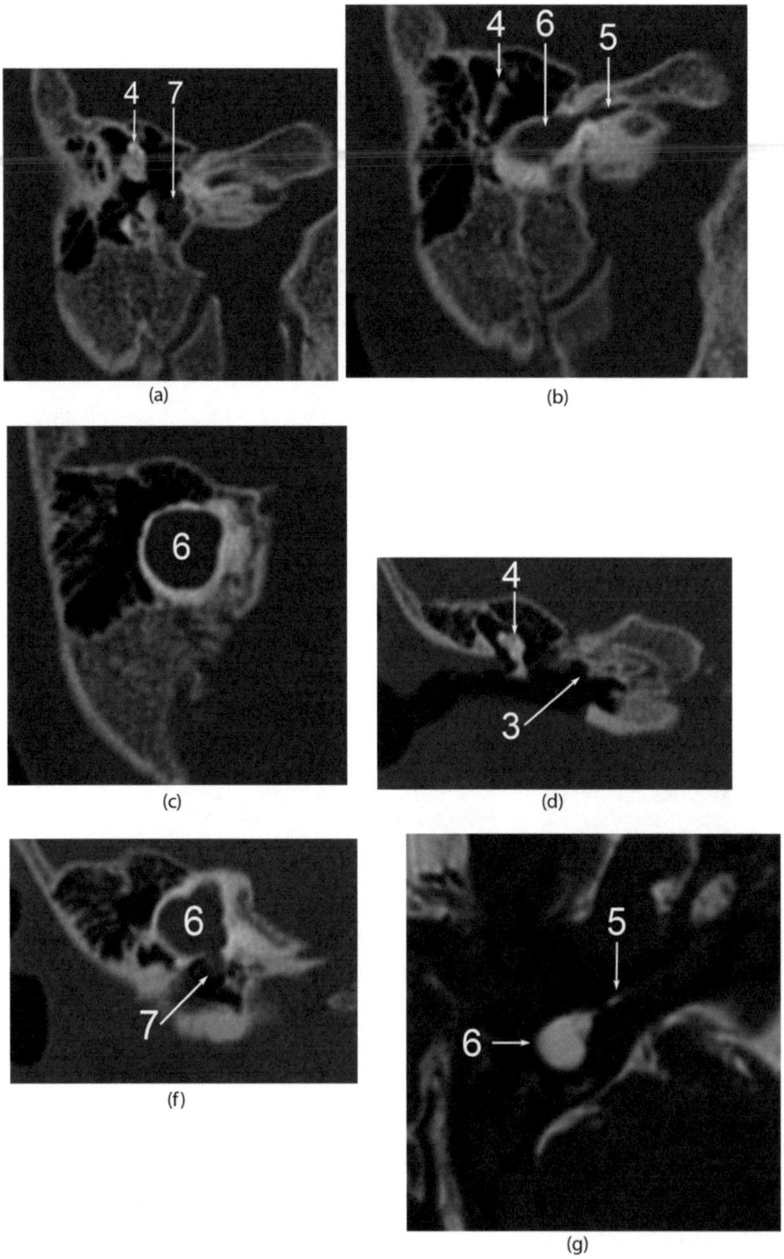

Figure 3.
(a–g) Young male T. Axial and coronary tomograms (CT and MRI) of the right temporal bone. 1—arch of the stirrup without footplate, 2—long process of the incus, 3—medial wall of the tympanic cavity, 4—anvil-malleolar complex, 5—internal auditory canal, 6—common cavity, 7—hernial-like protrusion of the lower sections of the common cavity into the tympanic cavity.

MRI of the brain and cochlear nerves. On the right—a common cavity 8x6.5 mm in size. The IAC is a narrow slit with a diameter of 0.5 mm. Neural structures are not visible (**Figure 3g**). On the left—a common cavity 3x2.5 mm in size. The IAC is

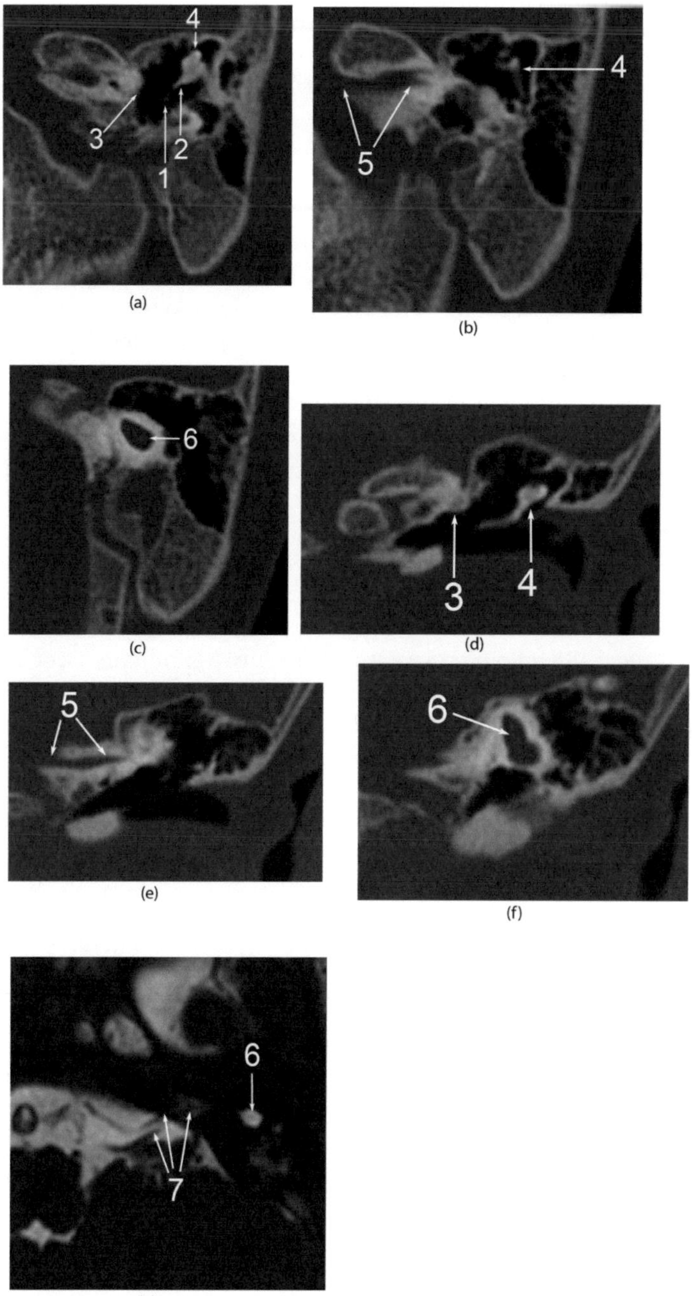

Figure 4.
(a–h) Young male T. Axial and coronary tomograms (CT and MRI) of the left temporal bone. 1—arch of the stirrup without footplate, 2—long process, 3—medial wall of the tympanic cavity, 4—incus-malleolar complex, 5—internal auditory canal, 6—common cavity and 7—neural structures in the internal auditory canal.

1.5x2.5 mm and contains cerebrospinal fluid, against which two neural structures (facial and undivided vestibulocochlear nerve) are traced, each up to 0.5 mm in diameter (**Figure 4g** and **h**).

Conclusion—MRI picture of aplasia of the vestibulocochlear nerve on the right and aplasia/hypoplasia on the left (caliber up to 0.5 mm) without signs of separation. Bilateral stenosis of the IAC. The council decided to perform cochlear implantation on the left ear. When the speech processor of the CI was first connected, a confident response to sounds was obtained, and further adjustments are being made.

5. Discussion

In the past decade, only one stenosis of the IAC, with a canal diameter of less than 1–2 mm, was considered a contraindication to CI. Currently, the indications for CT are expanding, and some children who previously belonged to absolutely unpromising children have moved into the group of potentially promising children, provided that the state of the anatomical structures of the temporal bone is correctly assessed. This was facilitated by the great technical progress of methods of radiation diagnostics. Thinner slices on CT and increased use of 3 T MRI have allowed for a finer level of evaluation of the anatomical structures of the temporal bone, especially the modiolus, cochlear aperture and cochlear nerve.

Conclusions: At present, stenosis of the IAC has ceased to be an absolute contraindication to CI. When determining the indications for CI and assessing its prospects in children with complex anomalies, it is necessary to comprehensively assess the state of all ear structures in CT and MR (preferably 3 T) images. In this case, the most critical is the state of the following structures: cochlea—modiolus—cochlear aperture—diameter of the IAC—the presence and condition of the cochlear nerve.

The absence of an image of the cochlear nerve (in the study of MRI 3 T) with complete bone obliteration of the cochlear aperture makes CI extremely unpromising.

In the presence of a normal or dysplastic cochlea, a hypoplastic cochlear nerve is not a contraindication for CI. In this situation, the presence of a modiolus and at least partially open cochlear aperture is prognostically favorable. Even in the case of hypoplasia of the cochlear nerve, the operation makes sense, and one can count on some success with this combination of anomalies.

Also, some clue pointing to the prospects of CI in severe anomalies of ear development can be the presence of certain hearing thresholds in a child before hearing falls to complete deafness.

In the presence of a large or small common cavity, an undivided vestibulocochlear nerve is not considered a contraindication for CI. Such a combination—a common cavity and an undivided vestibulocochlear nerve—is a prognostically quite favorable option.

Our results are encouraging and helpful in advising families on the likelihood of outcomes in relation to speech and auditory comprehension.

Conflict of interest

None.

Author details

Liia V. Toropchina[1*] and Elena I. Zelikovich[2]

1 FBSEI APE Russian Medical Academy of Continuous Professional Education of Ministry of Healthcare of Russia, Moscow, Russia

2 Moscow Health Department, L.I. Sverzhevsky Research Institute of Clinical Otorhinolaryngology, Moscow, Russia

*Address all correspondence to: liyatoropchina@yandex.ru

References

[1] Kari E, Go JL, Loggins J, Emmanuel N, Fisher LM. Abnormal Cochleovestibular anatomy and hearing outcomes: Pediatric patients with a questionable Cochleovestibular nerve status may Benefit from Cochlear implantation and/or hearing aids. Audiology & Neuro-Otology. 2018;**23**(1):48-57. DOI:10.1159/000488793

[2] Birman CS, Brew JA, Gibson WPR, Elliott EJ. CHARGE syndrome and Cochlear implantation: Difficulties and outcomes in the paediatric population. International Journal of Pediatric Otorhinolaryngology. 2015 Apr;**79**(4):487-492. DOI:10.1016/j.ijporl.2015.01.004

[3] Kari E, Gillard DM, Chuang N, Go JL. Can imaging predict hearing outcomes in children with Cochleovestibular nerve abnormalities? The Laryngoscope. 2022 Jun;**132**(Suppl 8):S1-S15. DOI:10.1002/lary.30008

[4] Chen JX, Nourmahnad A, O'Malley J, Reinshagen K Jr, Quesnel AM. Otopathology in CHARGE syndrome. Laryngoscope Investigative Otolaryngol. 2020;**5**(1):157-162. DOI:10.1002/lio2.347

[5] Hennersdorf F, Friese N, Löwenheim H, Tropitzsch A, Ernemann U, Bisdas S. Temporal bone changes in patients with Goldenhar syndrome with special emphasis on inner ear abnormalities. Otology & Neurotology. 2014;**35**(5):826-830. DOI:10.1097/MAO.0000000000000278

[6] Glastonbury CM, Davidson HC, Harnsberger HR, Butler J, Kertesz TR, Shelton C. Imaging findings of Cochlear nerve deficiency. AJNR. American Journal of Neuroradiology. 2002;**23**:635-643

Chapter 4

The Assessment of Electrode-Neuron Interface (ENI) in Cochlear Implant Users

Mohammad Maarefvand

Abstract

The electrode-neuron interface (ENI) plays an important in the outcome with cochlear implants as all cochlear implant-mediated signals should pass through this interface. Telemetry has enabled researchers to study factors affecting the quality and integrity of the interface. These factors may influence electrodes, the path between electrodes and auditory neurons, and spiral ganglion neuron survival. Promising studies on animals regarding such factors have opened new possibilities to identify cochlear implant channels with poor electrode-neuron interface. The results of these studies and similar research on human with focus were discussed in this chapter.

Keywords: cochlear implant, electrode-neuron interface, impedance, eCAP, SOE, phase duration, phase sensitivity, interphase gap, phase duration, mode of stimulation

1. Introduction

Cochlear implants (CIs) have been very successful in helping many people with severe to profound hearing loss to hear sounds and understand speech. However, some CI users cannot take enough benefits from these devices. To improve speech perception for all CI users, researchers have been trying to find the causes for such variability in speech perception. The said variability was observed among CI users of different devices manufactured by different companies. Therefore, it was reasonable to look into individual differences among CI users as the causes for the variability in speech perception. For example, research showed that CI users with better performance and speech perception had lost their hearing after language development. It means that they had reliable hearing in their early life (before age 2) [1]. Also, the early detection of hearing loss and less time interval between the detection and treatment were other factors that may contribute to better speech perception after using CIs along with lower age at the time of implantation [1]. The etiology of hearing loss could affect the performance since auditory neurons are significantly impaired in some etiologies of hearing loss more than other [1]. Although these factors can explain some differences in speech perception among CI users, most of the variability remains unexplained. Therefore, other reasons for individual differences should be sought.

Since the electrodes of CIs deliver speech information directly to auditory neurons, it is believed that the integrity of the meeting point of CI electrodes with the spiral ganglion neurons (SGNs) may influence the outcome with CIs. This meeting point is called the electrode-neuron interface (ENI). If the ENI is somehow impaired, the delivery of speech information is expected to be compromised. However, it is necessary to have an overview on how a typical CI works before further discussion about the ENI, which is the main topic of this chapter.

1.1 How does a CI work?

Although there are some differences in the design of CIs manufactured by different CI companies, the basic structure of all CI devices is similar. All CI devices have two parts: an external sound processor and internal receiver-stimulators connected to an electrode array. The external sound processors consist of three components. The first component is a microphone that picks up signals and converts them from acoustic to electric signals. The second component is a digital sound processor that analyzes the electrical signals into separate frequency bands. The signals are then converted into digital format and sent to the third component which is a transmitter. The transmitter is held in place by a magnet and sends the digitized information to the internal receiver-stimulator through radio frequency signals. The receiver-stimulator is a surgically implanted device in the mastoid bone, which is aligned with the transmitter through a magnet. The internal receiver-stimulator is attached to an electrode array and the electrode array is inserted into the scala tympani during surgery. The electrode array has different electrode contacts (up to 22). The receiver-stimulator decodes the received signals from the transmitter and sends these signals to its corresponding electrode contact within the cochlea. Each electrode inside the cochlea receives information about a limited range of frequency. Each electrode contact stimulates its adjacent auditory neurons electrically in a way that basal electrodes stimulate high-frequency SGNs and apical electrodes the low-frequency SGNs. The stimulated neurons convey the information from different electrodes to higher auditory centers and eventually to the auditory cortex for integration and sound perception [2].

1.2 Mode of stimulation

Cochlear implants work according to electricity principles. In electricity, electrical currents should flow in a circuit between two points. The active electrodes are the electrodes inside the cochlea (i.e., the scala tympani) which receive electric signals and stimulate the SGNs. To have a complete circuit, the signal delivered to the active electrodes should flow to a reference electrode. The reference electrode can be inside or outside the cochlea. For example, one of the adjacent electrodes close to the active electrode can be assigned as the reference electrode and can return the electrical current back to the receiver-stimulator. This mode of stimulation in called the bipolar mode (BP). In another mode, the intracochlear electrodes, which do not receive electrical stimulation, can be electronically connected together and return the stimulation delivered to the active electrode to receiver-stimulator. This mode of stimulation is called the common ground (CG). However, if the reference electrode is outside the cochlea, it can also receive the return current and this mode of stimulation is called the monopolar (MP). The path from receiver-stimulator to an active electrode and from an active electrode to its reference electrode and back to the receiver-stimulator forms a channel. Therefore, a channel consists of an active and a reference electrode [2].

The distance between active and reference electrodes in a channel determines the spread of electrical current to auditory neurons and the SGNs. In fact, MP modes produce the lowest thresholds for detection of sounds (T-levels) and comfortable level (C-levels) for speech perception [2]. As a result, the CIs with MP modes use less energy to produce stimulation, and have longer battery life. However, channel interaction (the interaction between the electrical fields produced around each active electrode) is more probable and pronounced with an MP mode [3]. Channel interaction can distort sound perception since this interaction may stimulate different overlapping populations of the SGNs at the same time and may reduce the resolution of stimulation. Despite this problem, MP modes are necessary for higher stimulation rates which are currently used in all CI devices and may result in better speech perception. In contrast, the shorter distance between active and reference electrodes in a BP mode may stimulate a limited neuron region and may lower the possibility of channel interactions but greater current is generally required to reach T- and C-levels. Due to the wider spread of current in a CG mode, this mode is basically similar to an MP mode. However, T- and C-levels in CG modes are usually higher than those levels in MP modes. One advantage of CG modes is that they can detect electrode anomalies which are discussed later in this chapter. One disadvantage of CG modes is that electrical current will flow to all electrodes including those outside the cochlea and could result in nonauditory percepts and it should not be used as a programming mode with CI recipients [2, 3].

1.3 Biphasic pulse

Regardless of the mode of stimulation, all current CI devices use biphasic pulses to stimulate auditory neurons. A biphasic pulse is a symmetrically charge-balanced stimulus. It means that negative (cathodic) and positive (anodic) phases are equal in terms of total charge, so that no net charge remains on auditory neurons after stimulation [3] and auditory neurons and the SGNs are stimulated safely with electrical pulses [3]. **Figure 1** shows an example of a typical biphasic pulse. A biphasic pulse has some characteristics. One of them is pulse width which is defined as the duration of each pulse in microseconds. The other one is current amplitude which is the amount of electrical current delivered to an active electrode. For a constant total charge, if pulse width is increased, current amplitude should decrease and vice versa [2, 3].

The total amount of charge delivered to neurons per phase of a biphasic current is equal to the product of current amplitude and pulse width: the greater the charge, the

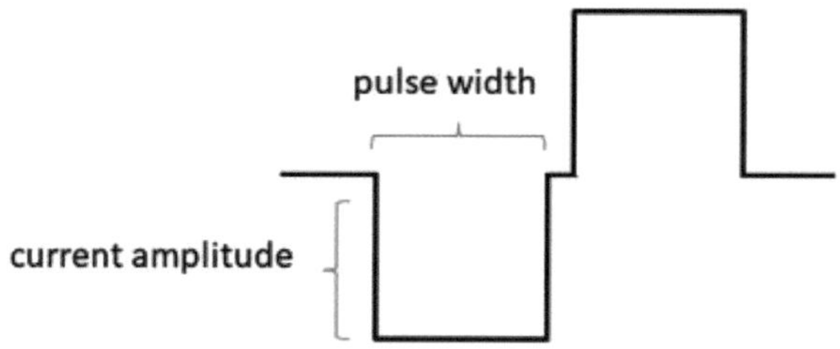

Figure 1.
Schematic representation of a typical biphasic pulse used for electrical stimulation of auditory neurons.

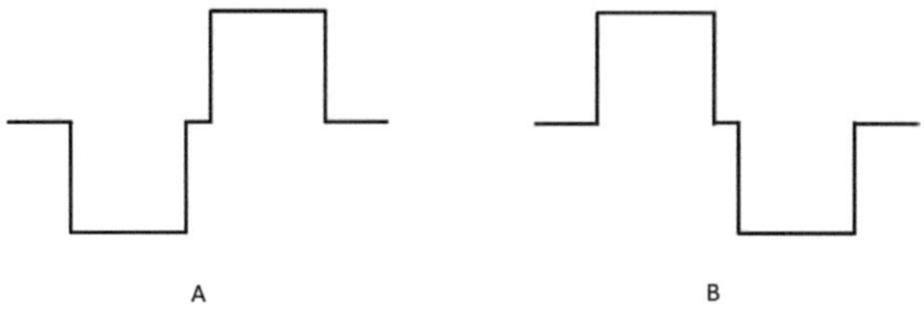

Figure 2.
Schematic representation of a negative-leading (A) and a positive-leading pulse (B).

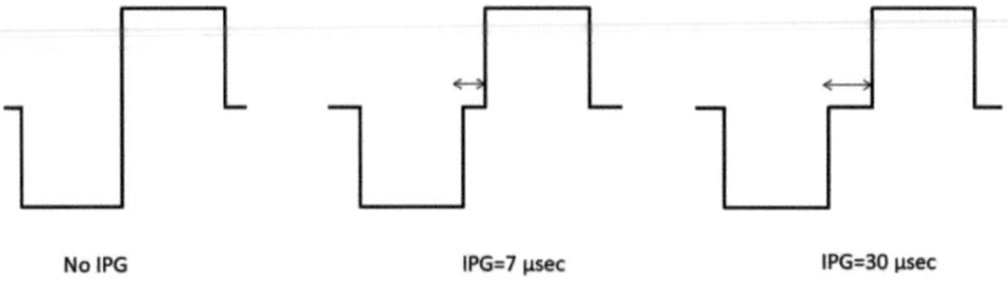

Figure 3.
Biphasic pulses with different interphase gap (IPG) lengths from zero (left) to 30 µs (right).

louder the sound. Increasing current amplitude or lengthening pulse width results in more charge and a louder sound. Biphasic pulses are presented in series to auditory neurons. They can be either negative-leading or positive-leading. If the first phase of a biphasic pulse is a negative phase, it is a negative-leading pulse and if the first phase of a biphasic pulse is a positive phase, it is a positive-leading pulse [2]. **Figure 2** shows the negative- and positive-leading pulses. By default, the stimulation of auditory neurons occurs during the negative phase of a biphasic pulse in current CIs by default.

Another characteristic of a biphasic signal is the interphase gap (IPG), which is the time interval between two phases of a biphasic signal. A biphasic pulse can vary from zero to as long as several hundred microoseconds. Different IPGs from 0 to 30 µs are shown schematically in **Figure 3**.

2. Factors affecting the ENI

Cochlear implant signals should go through a path from a CI electrode to reach its target neurons. The electrodes, path, and neurons can be impaired and such impairment potentially affects CI outcomes (i.e., speech and sound perception). For example, if CI electrodes are damaged, they cannot transmit sound signals to auditory neurons. Even when the CI electrodes are intact, but the location of the intact electrode is far from auditory neurons and SGNs, enough stimulation might not happen [2]. If an electrode and its location toward neurons are optimal but there are some physical obstacles between the electrode and neurons (such as bone growth and fibrous tissue), the strength of CI signals might be compromised or the signal might be diverted to unsuitable paths and could not reach the targeted neurons. Still when an electrode itself, its location relative to the neurons and the path are in ideal conditions, the auditory neurons and SGNs might be degenerated. Some etiologies or long duration of untreated deafness can degenerate or demyelinate auditory neurons and SGNs, and also reduce the size and number of SGNs survived after hearing loss [4]. Although there was not any significant correlation between the number of SGN numbers and speech perception [5], the quality of their functionality or the presence of auditory neurons' peripheral processes is an essential factor for proper perception by influencing the ENI [6, 7].

To assess the ENI, a test or batteries of tests are required to reveal information about each of the aforementioned factors. A better understanding of how the ENI influences outcomes will help to reduce damage during implantation, improve technology, and develop biologically fit therapies which can ultimately improve speech and sound perception. For example, if the ENI can be tested in human CI users and especially with clinical instruments, it may become clinically feasible to optimize CI programming parameters in a way that helps with better outcome in users who cannot take enough benefits from CI devices. Telemetry, using a radio frequency connection, has enabled CI devices for bidirectional communication of data. Simply, the external sound processor sends information to the implant and receives information back from the implant [2]. Several measurements take advantage of telemetry and they are now available in clinical software which can provide insights into the ENI. These measurements and recent findings are discussed below.

2.1 Impedance

Impedance testing is one of the applications of telemetry. In impedance testing, the opposition to electrical current flow in CI channels is assessed (i.e., opposition against electrical current flowing from receiver-stimulator to an active electrode and from active electrode to auditory neurons and then to the reference electrode). One way of impedance measurement is that a small electrical current is presented to a single active electrode [8]. Then, the required voltage to make the electrical current pass through the active electrode and travel back to the reference electrode is measured. Since at the reference electrode, both voltage and current values are known, it is possible to measure impedance for the active electrode using Ohm's law equation [Resistance (R) = Voltage (V)/Current (I)]. Higher the opposition, higher the voltage difference between the active and reference electrodes [8]. When a current is delivered to active electrodes, some factors resist the flow of an electrical current. The size and type of metal-forming wires and electrode contacts, the medium between electrodes and neurons, relative electrode position to the neurons, and the medium between active and reference electrodes all resist the flow of current in series. Therefore, their effects can be added together and presented as what is called the total access resistance. Reactance is another type of impedance that impedes current flow. Similar to a capacitor in which different plates hold positive and negative charges, the electrode surface and fluid/tissue hold opposing charges. The CI electrode surface acts as one of the capacitor plates and the fluid or tissue as another plate. They impede the flow of current by holding and storing electrical energy. Therefore, current can flow through the electrode surface to fluid/tissue with ions' movement rather than electron movements. The total impedance, in fact, is the vector sum of total access resistance and reactance [8].

Impedance tests are able to identify any break or discontinuity in the path of current from the source to the active electrodes and from active electrodes to the return electrodes in the MP mode. Any kind of break in this path results is very high impedance. This prevents proper neuron stimulation and most of time, they are deactivated by programming audiologists [2]. Another electrode anomaly may happen when two electrode contacts or the electrode wires come in touch with each other and they receive similar currents when only one of them is stimulated. These electrodes are short-circuited and their voltage difference will be close to zero. However, they will have normal impedance in MP modes in which the voltage difference is calculated between an intracochlear electrode and an out of cochlea reference electrode. However, when one of them is assigned to be active and another one to be the reference electrode (i.e., in CG and BP modes), their voltage difference is abnormally small [8].

Even when impedance values are within normal range, it is not guaranteed that the power source can deliver enough voltage to generate the required current levels. There are conditions in which even maximum voltage available from the implant is not enough to generate the required current level on an electrode. These conditions are called out of voltage compliance. The problem of out of voltage compliance may be due to increase in the impedance between electrode and neurons [8]. When this occurs, CI users do not perceive enough loudness with increase in stimulation level or loudness may fluctuate from time to time in line with variation in electrode impedance for a given current level [2].

There is another way that impedance can be measured with. In this way, a single active electrode is stimulated with a small current but the voltage difference is calculated for all combinations of intracochlear and reference electrodes. It means the voltage difference is measured between each intracochlear electrode and the extracochlear reference electrode while only one of the intracochlear electrodes (active electrode) receives stimulation. By definition, impedance is defined as opposition to "flow" of current. Therefore, there should be only measurable impedance (or voltage difference) between active intracochlear and extracochlear reference electrode. In reality, however, when an electrode receives stimulation, an electrical field may develop around it. This electrical field may spread to adjacent nonstimulated electrodes. As a result, there might be a voltage difference between nonstimulated and reference electrodes, even when they do not receive any electrical stimulation. However, impedance values for nonstimulated electrodes should be low compared to that of active electrode. Therefore, it is possible to create a matrix of voltage difference (or impedance) for all electrodes when only one active electrode receives stimulation. This matrix of voltage difference or its correspondence (i.e., impedance matrix) has been used to study current spread within the cochlea under different names (e.g., electrical field imaging and modeling [EFIM] or transimpedance matrix [TIM]) [8]. In addition to current spread, CI stimulation does not remain restricted to the targeted neurons and stimulates other overlapping neurons as well. This type of spread is called spread of neural excitation which is a physiological phenomenon and cannot be measured with impedance or voltage matrix since all types of impedance measurements deal with physical opposition to currents and physical current spread. The spread of neural excitation needs methods in which responses can be collected from stimulated neural population, which is discussed later in this chapter.

2.1.1 Impedance measurements for the assessment of the ENI

Clinically, it is possible to identify electrodes with short- and open-circuit anomalies with impedance testing. As these two anomalies can affect perception, the electrodes with these anomalies can be deactivated by clinicians. Also, electrodes with out of voltage compliance are detectable by current clinical applications. The out of voltage compliance might be a sign that the ENI is compromised [3, 8]. However, impedance assessment and voltage matrix can reveal more information about the

ENI. In one study on users of hybrid CI devices (i.e., a CI and hearing aid in the same ear), total impedance and access resistance were observed in two groups of users with stable and unstable residual hearing after implantation. Impedance values increased over time but the reactance component did not change in the group who experienced hearing loss after implantation. However, in the other group who had stable hearing after implantation, total impedance and access resistance were stable while reactance declined. The authors suggested that access resistance might be correlated with intracochlear fibrosis formation and inflammation in the ENI after surgery. The results were supported by animal study as well [9]. In addition, access resistance was reported to be able to detect translocation of the electrode arrays from scala tympani to scala vestibule [10].

Since one of the factors affecting the ENI might be the distance of electrodes from modiolus, impedance measures were found to be significantly higher for the perimodiolar array compared with straight arrays which are placed more distantly from modiolus [11, 12]. However, when the geometric electrode areas in the two arrays were normalized, there was not any difference in impedance values with the distance of electrodes relative to the modiolus. Behaviorally, electrode position within cochlea (lateral-wall versus medial-wall positioning) had significant correlation with audibility thresholds but could not predict speech perception [11–13]. While some studies reported association between speech perception and impedance results, two recently published studies on a large data set of CI users reject such a relationship [14, 15]. However, the variation in impedance values across the electrode array was significantly related to poorer speech recognition in both quiet and noise [14]. Different studies showed that the presence of obstacles in the ENI (such as fibrous and bone growth) might increase impedance and subsequently decrease cochlear implant function [16]. However, the negative effects of obstacles in the ENI are relatively unimportant in comparison to degeneration of auditory neurons and SGNs [17].

Voltage and TIM measurements have also shown a theoretical potential for evaluating electrode position [18]. However, there was not any strong association between the width of such matrices and behavioral assessments like speech perception in CI users with a full-insertion electrode array [19].

2.2 Electrical compound action potentials and neural health

One of the applications of telemetry is that, the neural responses can be gathered from auditory neurons and SGNs and are called electrical compound action potentials (eCAPs) in CI users. All contemporary CI software have the ability to generate and present electrical pulses to auditory neurons and then record neural responses [8]. These responses are then analyzed with computers and a waveform of the neural responses is depicted. Typically, a biphasic electrical pulse is presented to one active electrode and the neural responses arising from neurons are recorded via another electrode close (but not directly adjacent) to the active electrode. The separation between stimulated electrode (i.e., active electrode) and recording electrode will optimize the response amplitude while minimizing stimulus artifacts. The recorded responses are sent back to a computer via the external speech processor and a programming interface. The eCAP waveform typically consists of a negative deflection (N1), with the latency of 0.2–0.4 ms, followed by a positive peak (P2), with the latency of 0.5–0.7 ms [8].

The eCAP measurement can provide information regarding auditory neurons and SGN status: Three indices are usually calculated from eCAPs: threshold, amplitude-growth function (AGF), and amplitude. Therefore, these indices can be used as a means to assess the quality of the ENI. The threshold of eCAP is the lowest amount of current required for the recording of a measurable neural response. The response amplitude (measured in microvolts between N1 and P2) increases with increasing stimulus intensity. If the values of amplitudes of eCAP are depicted against current levels, an AGF is obtained. Also, the maximum amplitude of eCAP at or close to comfortable level can be calculated.

Since eCAPs are very short-latency responses, they may be obscured by transient electrical artifacts related to electrical pulses or amplifier saturation. To differentiate between real responses from electrical artifacts, the responses for a target stimulus (probe) are subtracted from responses for a masker in a forward-masking paradigm. Simply in this paradigm, pairs of maskers and probes are presented with a time interval and artifacts only affect neural responses to masker. However, the masker drives neurons into refractory period, a period in which auditory neurons physiologically do not respond to electric stimulation. The interval between the masker and probe is adjustable. By increase in this interval, more and more auditory neurons can recover from their refectory period and respond to the probe. More intervals between masker and probe, more contribution from the neurons recovered from refractory and therefore eCAP with larger amplitudes. After a specific interval (around 500 μs), all auditory neurons can respond to the probe and this response to the probe is an artifact-free response. The time interval required for responses from all neurons to probe may vary according to the health and integrity of auditory neurons. In fact, the recovery time represents the neural temporal responsiveness. The eCAPs measured with changing masker-probe interval or with fixed masker-probe interval have been used to study the ENI in several ways. The most relevant component of the ENI which is studied by eCAP is the neural health of auditory neurons and SGNs and the most studied aspect of neural health in human and animal has been the SGN density. The SGN density is quantified by the number of SGN cell bodies divided by the area containing those cell bodies in Rosenthal's canal [5].

In animal studies, the application of neomycin resulted in the total loss of SGNs along with other structural and functional damages to the cochlea. The amplitude, AGF slope of eCAP, and the latency of N1 were significantly correlated with the amount of SGN density [20, 21]. In guinea pigs receiving CIs, impairment to SGNs significantly lowered the speed of temporal recovery studied with eCAP masker-probe paradigm. In addition, the slopes of AGF declined over the first weeks after implantation and then recovered and became steeper and then stabilized. These changes are similar to the changes observed in behavioral detection measurements and they were attributed to inflammation in the cochlea after surgery. However, eCAP thresholds had poor correlation with behavioral threshold [22, 23] and did not reflect neural health [20].

In human studies, longer duration of hearing loss has been found to be associated with poor neural health [24]. Studies evaluating the association between the eCAP AGF slope and speech perception scores in human CI users show inconsistent results. Whereas, some studies reported better speech perception scores with sleeper slopes [25, 26], other studies found no association between these two measures [27, 28].

In addition, the eCAP AGF slope increased with increasing distance between the electrode and modiolus. A more recent study reported that the eCAP thresholds, but not necessarily eCAP AGF slope, were correlated with electrode-to-modiolus distance [29]. Hearing loss occurs differently in animal and human. In humans, some postmortem studies reported an overall decrease in SGN density in the ears with ossification, while other studies showed good SGN density in the ears with significant ossification [30, 31]. Specific etiologies of hearing loss (e.g., meningitis and sudden hearing losses caused by viral labyrinthitis) are also associated with the accumulation of tissue and bone formation in the scala tympani, even prior to the insertion of the cochlear implant electrode array [30]. One explanation for these contradictory findings could be related to the presence or absence of immune responses along with impairment to the inner ear. Concomitant presence of immune response and cochlear impairment could affect the density of SGNs as well as bone formation inside the cochlea.

2.2.1 ENI and SOE

In the assessment of the ENI, impedance and voltage matrices could give insights regarding the position of electrodes, bony or fibrous tissue formation, and current spread inside the cochlea. However, the spread of physical current per se cannot provide information about the physiological spread of neural excitation. It is assumed that when current spread is wide, more auditory neurons and SGNs in the wider area would be stimulated and current spread and neural excitation spread are correlated. However, studies showed that the spread of neural excitation might not always be reflected in the current spread assessed by voltage or TIM [18, 32]. Therefore, both current spread and spread of neural activation should be measured in the thorough assessment of the ENI, as they both may reduce the neural resolution of CI stimulation and subsequently the perception of sounds.

Electrical compound action potential can be used to provide information regarding the spread of neural activation. Using forward-masking paradigm, an active electrode is stimulated and eCAP amplitudes are measured for that electrode and the electrodes adjacent to it. A function of eCAP amplitudes for active and adjacent electrodes is formed, which may show the spread of excitation (SOE) of auditory neurons and SGNs. In this measurement, the probe electrode is presented to the active electrode and variable maskers to adjacent electrodes [8]. The separation in the location of the probe and maskers may provide eCAP amplitude from different neuron regions around the active electrode. Ideally, the maximum amplitude of eCAP should belong to neuron stimulated by the active electrode with much lower amplitudes from neurons stimulated by adjacent electrodes. However, the overlap between different neuronal populations may create wide SOE function. The width of the SOE function is calculated and reveals information about the amount of overlap between different neuron regions in responding to electrical stimulation (i.e., spread of neural excitation) [2, 8].

Some studies have shown that current spread and spread of neural excitation were not significantly correlated [18]. For example, the results of TIM and SOE were not related, except for a middle electrode [33]. In contrast to early studies which claimed that close distance between electrodes and spiral ganglion would result in a narrow current spread, there was not any significant difference in SOE widths for perimodiolar versus straight electrode array [34]. Although, SOE could help with intraoperative identification of abnormalities of intracochlear electrodes (such as folded electrodes), the computerized tomography (CT) is the ideal test for a precise determination of the position and location of the electrodes within cochlear.

When the relationship of the SOE width and behavioral tests (e.g., speech and pitch discrimination) was studied, there was not any significant correlation between them [35, 36]. However, it should be taken into consideration that speech perception is assessed with stimulation of a wide range of intracochlear electrodes while the SOE width is calculated from the stimulation of few intracochlear electrodes and this might partially justify the lack of correlation between eCAP SOE width and speech perception outcome [35, 36]. Moreover, speech perception is influenced by central auditory processing which is not assessed by the SOE. Therefore, the eCAP SOE function should not be used as the sole objective measure for predicting speech perception in CI users. However, this measure may provide useful information about channel interaction and the possibility of neural dead region which might influence the ENI and CI outcome.

2.2.2 ENI and recovery time

Intuitively, it is believed that faster recovery from refractory period is related to more efficient neural response and better neural health than slower recovery. In fact, faster recovery from refractoriness has been reported to correlate with better speech perception scores in some studies [23, 37, 38]. However, this association was not observed in other studies [28, 39, 40]. Even when recovery time was compared between single and large numbers of neurons, slower recovery from refractory period was associated with greater temporal responsiveness, which was a manifestation of larger neural population and better neural health.

Two phases of refractory period have been identified in studies on auditory neurons and SGNs. The first phase is the absolute refractory period in which the auditory neurons cannot be stimulated even with very intense stimuli. The second phase of the refractory period is called relative refractory period in which auditory neurons can be activated by intense stimuli. However, the speed of recovery from refractoriness is affected by stimulus level, with faster recovery at higher levels [41].

The effect of advanced age on the recovery time from refractory was assessed in postlingually middle-aged adult and elderly CI users using eCAP. There was faster recovery at higher pulse rates and for longer durations of stimulation. There was no significant effect of age on the speed of recovery from refractory period [39, 40].

In another study based on measuring refractory recovery, there were no significant age group differences in refractory times, eCAP thresholds, and N1 latencies. However, the slopes of the eCAP AGF were significantly larger in the middle-aged group compared to the elderly group. Except for N1 latency, electrode location significantly influenced eCAP [39].

Several studies have investigated the refractory properties of the auditory neurons and SGNs in people with special conditions such as the auditory neuropathy spectrum disorder (ANSD) and cochlear nerve deficiency [23]. Children with ANSD had similar refractory recovery time compared with children with typical sensorineural hearing loss [37]. Children with cochlear nerve deficiency had longer absolute refractory time compared with implanted children with normal-sized auditor nerve, but two groups had similar relative refractory [23]. However, the relative refractory period was longer in people with longer duration of hearing loss [39, 42]. There was no difference in the temporal recovery of the auditory nerve between pre- and postlingual CI users [43].

2.2.3 ENI and pulse duration

Animal studies showed that auditory neurons and SGN density were sensitive to changes in parameters of stimulation signals such as increase in pulse duration [20].

Basically, the total amount of charges delivered to auditory neurons will increase when the duration of a biphasic pulse increases. If the auditory neurons are healthy, more current is integrated at the cell membrane and stronger eCAP can be recorded with increase in pulse duration. Therefore, eCAP elicited with different pulse durations has the potential to assess auditory neural health and to be a means for the assessment of the ENI.

The threshold, slope of AGF, and amplitude of eCAP were recorded after changing biphasic pulse duration and interphase gap and the results were correlated with histological and behavioral evidence in guinea pigs receiving CIs. The threshold of eCAP decreased with increase in duration and interphase gap while both amplitude and slope increased. However, the histological findings and eCAP were not correlated [20, 44].

In a human study, the pulse duration was increased in two groups of children using CIs. One group had normal cochlear nerve size and the other group had deficiency in cochlear nerve. The eCAP results showed that increase in duration from 50 to 88 μs did not significantly change cochlear nerve responsiveness to electrical stimulation in either group for a biphasic pulse in MP mode when electrical charge was kept constant [23].

2.2.4 *ENI and phase sensitivity*

Animal and modeling studies have shown that if the values of eCAP measures are very different for negative- and positive-leading biphasic signals, it theoretically reflects poorer neural health, whereas smaller differences indicate better neural health [45–47]. In healthy auditory neurons, both negative- and positive-leading pulses activate peripheral processes and initiate spikes at threshold level. At high stimulus level, the negative-leading pulses still stimulate peripheral processes, whereas positive-leading pulses inhibit peripheral processes and generate spikes at cell body.

In cases where peripheral processes are degenerated, the only site that can generate neural spikes is cell body by negative-leading stimuli. Compared with the peripheral axon, the cell body has a much higher threshold, which results in a higher threshold for negative-leading stimuli while the response of the cell body to positive-leading stimuli at high stimulus levels is not affected. As a result, at an equal stimulus level, negative-leading pulses are more effective at generating a neural response from intact human auditory nerve fibers, whereas positive-leading pulses are more effective when peripheral processes are absent or demyelinated [47]. Therefore, comparing the difference in eCAP evoked by two types of pulses may provide useful information about neural survival of auditory nerve fibers [48].

Changing polarity has been used to assess neural health as one of the factors affecting the ENI. They showed at a fixed stimulus level, eCAP evoked by positive-leading biphasic pulses elicited larger amplitudes, shorter latencies, and steeper AGF slopes than those evoked by negative-leading biphasic pulses [48]. These results indicated the possibility of degeneration of the peripheral processes in the deaf ears [49]. However, the association between speech perception capability and polarity sensitivity has not been evaluated in a human CI user. Higher threshold levels were reported for poor neural health in human when they were tested with focused stimulation and the thresholds were not influenced by the position of electrodes inside the cochlea and resistance against current flow [50]. The CI adults with long duration of deafness and poor neural health had better sensitivity to anodic pulses but this was not observed in children using CIs [45].

2.2.5 ENI and IPG change

It is believed that increase in the interphase gap of a biphasic signal allows auditory neurons and SGNs to better recover from depolarization if auditory neurons are in healthy condition. With increase in IPG, lower threshold, steeper AGF slope, and higher amplitude are expected for eCAP. Smaller changes in these measures are observed when auditory neurons and SGNs are degenerated. The IPG effect is thought to be dependent on membrane characteristics, and thus reflect the temporal response properties of the auditory nerve [51]. Given that the IPG effect is a measure performed within the same channel or electrode, it should be less influenced by nonneural conditions that vary across the electrode array (e.g., electrode impedance, fibrous growth, and electrode position) [52]. Compared with fixed IPG, eCAP recorded for different IPG can reveal more information about auditory neuron health.

In animals, the sensitivity to IPG has been shown to be predictive of SGN density. For example, guinea pigs with lower densities of SGNs showed larger IPG effects on the eCAP threshold, amplitude, and N1 latency while in human, the IPG effect was observed for the slope of the AGF [20, 44]. However, IPG effect assessed in animals showed different results from those measured in human CI users.

In a human study on two groups of child CI users with normal-sized and deficient cochlear nerves, the IPG effect showed itself to be in larger amplitude and slope of AGF of eCAP and smaller on the eCAP threshold and N1 latency [53]. However, there was smaller increase in amplitude and slope of AGF eCAP along with higher eCAP threshold in children with nerve deficiency. The effect of increasing IPG from 7 to 30 μs has been studied in another study on CI users. It was shown that increasing IPG generally yielded increased eCAP amplitude and steeper slopes of AGF. However, this effect varied across subjects and electrode locations [24].

It is assumed that SGN density may vary as a function of age at implantation and hearing loss etiology. This assumption was studied on two groups of people who were implanted at early age and adulthood while IPG increased. The group who were implanted at early age had larger changes in eCAP amplitude. However, the AGF slope and eCAP threshold did not differ between the two groups. Irrespective of IPG, child-implanted participants had larger eCAP amplitudes and steeper AGF slopes than the adult-implanted participants. However, vowel recognition performance was not significantly correlated with any of the eCAP measures assessed in this study.

2.2.6 ENI and mode of stimulation

The MP mode creates a relatively broad spread of current. More restricted current spread can be achieved with focused stimulation modes, in which current delivered to an active electrode is returned to the source through "adjacent intracochlear electrodes" or a "combination of adjacent intracochlear and extracochlear reference electrodes." These focused stimulation modes likely stimulate a more localized region of the auditory neurons and SGNs and can be more sensitive to localized neural degeneration of auditory neurons and reduction in SGNs. Therefore, these focused stimulations have potential for the assessment of neural health and the ENI.

Focused stimulation modes have been used in electrophysiological and behavioral assessment of the ENI. Younger CI users are assumed to have better auditory neurons and SGNs than older CI users. When eCAP was used to capture neural responses to focused stimulation in these two groups, young CI users had steeper eCAP AGF slopes and larger amplitudes and they showed more sensitivity to changes in IPG. In another study, child-implanted CI users had steeper AGF slopes and larger amplitudes compared to adult-implanted CI users. The IPG effect for eCAP amplitude was significant but not for slope or threshold [54].

In another study, behavioral thresholds using focused stimulation were determined across channels. The high and low threshold channels in focused stimulation were considered as channels with poor and good ENI, respectively [6]. Using eCAP measurements, the high-threshold channels had higher eCAP thresholds, steeper AGF slopes than low-threshold channels. In another study, subjects with low-focused behavioral thresholds showed large eCAP amplitudes. Higher speech perception scores had significant correlation with low-focused thresholds [55].

Also, the polarity of pulse signals was changed (polarity effect) in focused stimulation studies and the results indicated that the polarity effect was not related to non-neural factors such as electrode-to-modiolus distance, electrode location inside the cochlea, or resistance. In fact, positive polarity effects, which may indicate SGN degeneration, were associated with relatively high focused behavioral thresholds. Overall, these results provide support for the theory that the polarity effect may reflect neural integrity in CI listeners.

2.2.7 ENI and other behavioral tests

In addition to objective measures, some behavioral testing measures have been tried for the assessment of the ENI. One of them is the multipulse integration (MPI) test, in which the difference between thresholds at different rate is calculated. MPI refers to a decrease (improvement) in the psychophysical detection threshold with increasing pulse rate of CI stimulation while the duration of pulse trains remains constant. MPI slopes are calculated as the amount of threshold decrease per increase in pulse rate. This slope is calculated for pulse rates over a range from a few up to about 1000 pulses per second (pps) [56].

Studies on animals have shown that the slope of the MPI function differs between animals with lower and higher SGN densities [17, 57–61], but only in animals with preserved IHCs [10]. In another behavioral test, temporal integration was assessed with the determination of detection thresholds for constant pulse rates varying in duration. The results showed correlation with cochlear health [58].

The behavioral threshold changes can be measured for changing in pulse phase duration in experiments, which are referred to as strength-duration function tests. The slope (changes in thresholds for changing duration) of the function is considered as a predictor for variations in cochlear health [62]. The characteristics of strength-duration functions can be influenced with the degeneration of the peripheral processes. If these processes are degenerated, the site of neural spike generation is shifted from peripheral neurons to more central axonal regions that have better myelination [63]. It was shown that psychophysical strength-duration function slopes were significantly shallower in guinea pigs implanted in an ear with residual hearing compared with those implanted in a deafened ear that was treated with neurotrophin. In animals deafened with neomycin and treated with neurotrophin, which typically had no surviving inner hair cells, the slopes of the psychophysical strength-duration functions were correlated with spiral ganglion neuron (SGN) density, being steeper in cases with higher SGN densities. However, in animals implanted in a hearing ear, which typically had surviving inner hair cells, slopes of the strength-duration functions were not correlated with SGN density. In addition, the strength-duration slopes were not predictive of duration of any hearing loss or speech recognition performance.

3. Conclusion

Many factors exist that influence the outcome with CI devices by influencing the ENI. Some of them, which could be assessed clinically, were discussed in this chapter. However, there are other factors, such as residual hearing preservation, the type and dimension of electrode arrays and their insertion depth, which are important. In addition, since speech performance needs the processing of sounds in the central auditory system, this factor and cognitive ability of a CI user impact speech perception with CIs. These factors were out of the scope of this chapter, as the focus of this chapter was on the assessments which can be performed with clinically available applications.

There was some discrepancy between animal and human findings, which may stem from different etiologies and pattern of hearing loss in human CI users. There were also differences in the research methods between the two species. It seems that a battery test of current clinical application can be used in the assessment of the ENI. However, the findings of these tests should have well-established association with behavioral findings which needs more controlled studies.

Author details

Mohammad Maarefvand
Department of Audiology, Iran University of Medical Sciences, Tehran, Iran

*Address all correspondence to: maarefvandm@gmail.com

References

[1] Lazard DS, Vincent C, Venail F, Van de Heyning P, Truy E, Sterkers O, et al. Pre-, per- and postoperative factors affecting performance of postlinguistically deaf adults using cochlear implants: A new conceptual model over time. PLoS One. 2012;**7**(11):1-11

[2] Wolfe J. Cochlear Implants: Audiologic Management and Considerations for Implantable Hearing Devices. San Diego, CA: Plural Publishing, Incorporated; 2018

[3] Litovsky RY, Goupell MJ, Kan A, Landsberger DM. Use of research interfaces for psychophysical studies with cochlear-implant users. Trends in Hearing. 2017;**21**:1-15

[4] Seyyedi M, Viana LM, Nadol JB Jr. Within-subject comparison of word recognition and spiral ganglion cell count in bilateral cochlear implant recipients. Otology & Neurotology. 2014;**35**(8):1446-1450

[5] Cheng Y-S, Svirsky MA. Meta-analysis—Correlation between spiral ganglion cell counts and speech perception with a cochlear implant. Audiology Research. 2021;**11**(2):220-226

[6] Bierer JA. Probing the electrode-neuron interface with focused cochlear implant stimulation. Trends in Amplification. 2010;**14**(2):84-95

[7] Schvartz-Leyzac KC, Colesa DJ, Swiderski DL, Raphael Y, Pfingst BE. Cochlear health and cochlear-implant function. Journal of the Association for Research in Otolaryngology. 2023;**24**(1):5-29

[8] Hughes ML. Objective Measures in Cochlear Implants. San Diego, CA: Plural Pub; 2013

[9] Tykocinski M, Cohen LT, Pyman BC, Roland T Jr, Treaba C, Palamara J, et al. Comparison of electrode position in the human cochlea using various perimodiolar electrode arrays. Otology & Neurotology. 2000;**21**(2):205-211

[10] Dong Y, Briaire JJ, Siebrecht M, Stronks HC, Frijns JHM. Detection of translocation of cochlear implant electrode arrays by intracochlear impedance measurements. Ear and Hearing. 2021;**42**(5):1397-1404

[11] Degen CV, Büchner A, Kludt E, Lenarz T. Effect of electrode to modiolus distance on electrophysiological and psychophysical parameters in ci patients with perimodiolar and lateral electrode arrays. Otology & Neurotology. 2020;**41**(9):e1091-e1097

[12] Long CJ, Holden TA, McClelland GH, Parkinson WS, Shelton C, Kelsall DC, et al. Examining the electro-neural interface of cochlear implant users using psychophysics, ct scans, and speech understanding. Journal of the Association for Research in Otolaryngology. 2014;**15**(2):293-304

[13] Zarowski A, Molisz A, Cardinael E, Vermeiren A, Theunen T, De Coninck L, et al. Prediction of behavioral t/c levels in cochlear implant patients based upon analysis of electrode impedances. Journal of the American Academy of Audiology. 2020;**31**(9):674-679

[14] de Graaff F, Lissenberg-Witte BI, Kaandorp MW, Merkus P, Goverts ST, Kramer SE, et al. Relationship between speech recognition in quiet and noise and fitting parameters, impedances and ecap thresholds in adult cochlear implant users. Ear and Hearing. 2020;**41**(4):935-947

[15] Pisa JFD, Almutairi WH, Mackie K, Stangherlin D, Sulkers J, Hochman JB. Impedance change as an indicator of cochlear implant failure. Otology & Neurotology. 2023;**44**(4):e211-e215

[16] Wilk M, Hessler R, Mugridge K, Jolly C, Fehr M, Lenarz T, et al. Impedance changes and fibrous tissue growth after cochlear implantation are correlated and can be reduced using a dexamethasone eluting electrode. PLoS One. 2016;**11**(2):e0147552

[17] Swiderski DL, Colesa DJ, Hughes AP, Raphael Y, Pfingst BE. Relationships between intrascalar tissue, neuron survival, and cochlear implant function. Journal of the Association for Research in Otolaryngology. 2020;**21**(4):337-352

[18] Söderqvist S, Lamminmäki S, Aarnisalo A, Hirvonen T, Sinkkonen ST, Sivonen V. Intraoperative transimpedance and spread of excitation profile correlations with a lateral-wall cochlear implant electrode array. Hearing Research. 2021;**405**:108235

[19] Swaddiwudhipong N, Jiang C, Landry TG, Bance M. Investigating the electrical properties of different cochlear implants. Otology & Neurotology. 2021;**42**(1):59-67

[20] Ramekers D, Versnel H, Strahl SB, Smeets EM, Klis SFL, Grolman W. Auditory-nerve responses to varied inter-phase gap and phase duration of the electric pulse stimulus as predictors for neuronal degeneration. Journal of the Association for Research in Otolaryngology. 2014;**15**(2):187-202

[21] Ramekers D, Benav H, Klis SFL, Versnel H. Changes in the electrically evoked compound action potential over time after implantation and subsequent deafening in Guinea pigs. Journal of the Association for Research in Otolaryngology. 2022;**23**(6):721-738

[22] Jeon EK, Brown CJ, Etler CP, O'Brien S, Chiou L-K, Abbas PJ. Comparison of electrically evoked compound action potential thresholds and loudness estimates for the stimuli used to program the advanced bionics cochlear implant. Journal of the American Academy of Audiology. 2010;**21**(01):016-027

[23] He S, Teagle HFB, Buchman CA. The electrically evoked compound action potential: From laboratory to clinic. Frontiers in Neuroscience. 2017;**11**:339

[24] Schvartz-Leyzac KC, Pfingst BE. Across-site patterns of electrically evoked compound action potential amplitude-growth functions in multichannel cochlear implant recipients and the effects of the interphase gap. Hearing Research. 2016;**341**:50-65

[25] Schvartz-Leyzac KC, Pfingst BE. Assessing the relationship between the electrically evoked compound action potential and speech recognition abilities in bilateral cochlear implant recipients. Ear and Hearing. 2018;**39**(2):344-358

[26] Dong Y, Briaire JJ, Stronks HC, Frijns JHM. Speech perception performance in cochlear implant recipients correlates to the number and synchrony of excited auditory nerve fibers derived from electrically evoked compound action potentials. Ear and Hearing. 2023;**44**(2):276-286

[27] Langner F, Arenberg JG, Büchner A, Nogueira W. Assessing the relationship between neural health measures and speech performance with simultaneous electric stimulation in cochlear implant listeners. PLoS One. 2021;**16**(12):1-21

[28] Turner C, Mehr M, Hughes M, Brown C, Abbas P. Within-subject predictors of speech recognition in cochlear implants: A null result. Acoustics Research Letters Online. 2002;**3**(3):95-100

[29] Imsiecke M, Büchner A, Lenarz T, Nogueira W. Amplitude growth functions of auditory nerve responses to electric pulse stimulation with varied interphase gaps in cochlear implant users with ipsilateral residual hearing. Trends in Hearing. 2021;**25**:1-15

[30] Green JD Jr, Marion MS, Hinojosa R. Labyrinthitis ossificans: Histopathologic consideration for cochlear implantation. Otolaryngology and Head and Neck Surgery. 1991;**104**(3):320-326

[31] Nadol JB, Hsu W. Histopathologic correlation of spiral ganglion cell count and new bone formation in the cochlea following meningogenic labyrinthitis and deafness. The Annals of Otology, Rhinology, and Laryngology. 1991;**100**(9):712-716

[32] Kopsch AC, Rahne T, Plontke SK, Wagner L. Influence of the spread of electric field on neural excitation in cochlear implant users: Transimpedance and spread of excitation measurements. Hearing Research. 2022;**424**:108591

[33] Bierer JA, Faulkner KF. Identifying cochlear implant channels with poor electrode-neuron interface: Partial tripolar, single-channel thresholds and psychophysical tuning curves. Ear and Hearing. 2010;**31**(2):247-258

[34] Kalkman RK, Briaire JJ, Frijns JH. Current focussing in cochlear implants: An analysis of neural recruitment in a computational model. Hearing Research. 2015;**322**:89-98

[35] van der Beek FB, Briaire JJ, Frijns JHM. Effects of parameter manipulations on spread of excitation measured with electrically-evoked compound action potentials. International Journal of Audiology. 2012;**51**(6):465-474

[36] Cohen LT, Richardson LM, Saunders E, Cowan RSC. Spatial spread of neural excitation in cochlear implant recipients: Comparison of improved ecap method and psychophysical forward masking. Hearing Research. 2003;**179**(1):72-87

[37] Fulmer SL, Runge CL, Jensen JW, Friedland DR. Rate of neural recovery in implanted children with auditory neuropathy spectrum disorder. Otolaryngology and Head and Neck Surgery. 2011;**144**(2):274-279

[38] Kiefer J, Hohl S, Stürzebecher E, Pfennigdorff T, Gstöettner W. Comparison of speech recognition with different speech coding strategies (SPEAK, CIS, and ACE) and their relationship to telemetric measures of compound action potentials in the nucleus CI 24m cochlear implant system. Audiology. 2001;**40**(1):32-42

[39] Lee ER, Friedland DR, Runge CL. Recovery from forward masking in elderly cochlear implant users. Otology & Neurotology. 2012;**33**(3):355-363

[40] Skidmore J, Carter BL, Riggs WJ, He S. The effect of advanced age on the electrode-neuron interface in cochlear implant users. Ear and Hearing. 2022;**43**(4):1300-1315

[41] Finley CC, Holden TA, Holden LK, Whiting BR, Chole RA, Neely GJ, et al. Role of electrode placement as a contributor to variability in cochlear implant outcomes. Otology & Neurotology. 2008;**29**(7):920-928

[42] Botros A, Psarros C. Neural response telemetry reconsidered: II. The influence

of neural population on the ecap recovery function and refractoriness. Ear and Hearing. 2010;**31**(3):380-391

[43] Carvalho B, Wiemes GRM, Patrial Netto L, Hamerschmidt R. Neural recovery function of the auditory nerve in cochlear implant surgery: Comparison between prelingual and postlingual patients. International Archives of Otorhinolaryngology. 2020;**24**:e444-e449

[44] Prado-Guitierrez P, Fewster LM, Heasman JM, McKay CM, Shepherd RK. Effect of interphase gap and pulse duration on electrically evoked potentials is correlated with auditory nerve survival. Hearing Research. 2006;**215**(1):47-55

[45] Jahn KN, Arenberg JG. Polarity sensitivity in pediatric and adult cochlear implant listeners. Trends in Hearing. 2019;**23**:1-22

[46] Joshi SN, Dau T, Epp B. A model of electrically stimulated auditory nerve fiber responses with peripheral and central sites of spike generation. Journal of the Association for Research in Otolaryngology. 2017;**18**(2):323-342

[47] Resnick JM, O'Brien GE, Rubinstein JT. Simulated auditory nerve axon demyelination alters sensitivity and response timing to extracellular stimulation. Hearing Research. 2018;**361**:121-137

[48] Undurraga JA, Carlyon RP, Macherey O, Wouters J, van Wieringen A. Spread of excitation varies for different electrical pulse shapes and stimulation modes in cochlear implants. Hearing Research. 2012;**290**(1):21-36

[49] Fayad JN, Linthicum FH Jr. Multichannel cochlear implants: Relation of histopathology to performance. The Laryngoscope. 2006;**116**(8):1310-1320

[50] Jahn KN, Arenberg JG. Evaluating psychophysical polarity sensitivity as an indirect estimate of neural status in cochlear implant listeners. Journal of the Association for Research in Otolaryngology. 2019;**20**(4):415-430

[51] van den Honert C, Mortimer JT. The response of the myelinated nerve fiber to short duration biphasic stimulating currents. Annals of Biomedical Engineering. 1979;**7**(2):117-125

[52] Schvartz-Leyzac KC, Holden TA, Zwolan TA, Arts HA, Firszt JB, Buswinka CJ, et al. Effects of electrode location on estimates of neural health in humans with cochlear implants. Journal of the Association for Research in Otolaryngology. 2020;**21**(3):259-275

[53] Skidmore J, He S. The effect of increasing interphase gap on n1 latency of the electrically evoked compound action potential and the stimulation level offset in human cochlear implant users. Ear and Hearing. 2020;**42**(1):244-247

[54] Jahn KN, Arenberg JG. Electrophysiological estimates of the electrode–neuron interface differ between younger and older listeners with cochlear implants. Ear and Hearing. 2020;**41**(4):948-960

[55] DiNino M, O'Brien G, Bierer SM, Jahn KN, Arenberg JG. The estimated electrode-neuron interface in cochlear implant listeners is different for early-implanted children and late-implanted adults. Journal of the Association for Research in Otolaryngology. 2019;**20**(3):291-303

[56] Zhou N, Dong L, Hang M. Evaluating multipulse integration as a neural-health correlate in human cochlear implant users: Effects of stimulation mode. Journal of the Association for Research in Otolaryngology. 2018;**19**(1):99-111

[57] Kang SY, Colesa DJ, Swiderski DL, Su GL, Raphael Y, Pfingst BE. Effects of hearing preservation on psychophysical responses to cochlear implant stimulation. Journal of the Association for Research in Otolaryngology. 2010;**11**(2):245-265

[58] Pfingst BE, Bowling SA, Colesa DJ, Garadat SN, Raphael Y, Shibata SB, et al. Cochlear infrastructure for electrical hearing. Hearing Research. 2011;**281**(1):65-73

[59] Pfingst BE, Colesa DJ, Hembrador S, Kang SY, Middlebrooks JC, Raphael Y, et al. Detection of pulse trains in the electrically stimulated cochlea: Effects of cochlear health. The Journal of the Acoustical Society of America. 2011;**130**(6):3954-3968

[60] Pfingst BE, Colesa DJ, Swiderski DL, Hughes AP, Strahl SB, Sinan M, et al. Neurotrophin gene therapy in deafened ears with cochlear implants: Long-term effects on nerve survival and functional measures. Journal of the Association for Research in Otolaryngology. 2017;**18**(6):731-750

[61] Zhou N, Kraft CT, Colesa DJ, Pfingst BE. Integration of pulse trains in humans and Guinea pigs with cochlear implants. Journal of the Association for Research in Otolaryngology. 2015;**16**(4):523-534

[62] Abbas PJ, Hughes ML, Brown CJ, Miller CA, South H. Channel interaction in cochlear implant users evaluated using the electrically evoked compound action potential. Audiology & Neuro-Otology. 2004;**9**(4):203-213

[63] Javel E, Shepherd RK. Electrical stimulation of the auditory nerve: Iii. Response initiation sites and temporal fine structure. Hearing Research. 2000;**140**(1):45-76

Section 2

CI Hearing Rehabilitation Strategies

Chapter 5

Anatomy-Based Programming

Isra Aljazeeri, Yassin Abdelsamad and Abdulrahman Hagr

Abstract

The ultimate goal of a cochlear implant device is to mimic the hearing through normal cochlea. A better understanding of normal cochlear function can help reaching this goal. The normal cochlea has a tonotopic mapping of the frequency representation in which each area on the cochlea is the most sensitive to a specific frequency. The array of the cochlear implant device has a number of electrodes each presenting a different frequency to the nearest area of the cochlea to where they are located. An anatomy-based programming strategy aims to present the frequency by the electrode contacts to which the cochlea is most sensitive to, according to the location of that electrode contact inside the cochlea. This chapter explores the details of the current understanding of the anatomy-based programming.

Keywords: cochlea, anatomy, anatomy-based, programming, fitting, frequency-to-place mismatch

1. Introduction

Cochlear implant device is one of the most successful invented implants. It is used in patients who have lost their hearing sensation and have sensorineural hearing loss. The cochlear implant device has an external part containing a microphone and speech processor and an internal part that is implanted surgically and contains an internal receiver stimulator and an electrode array. The internal part of the multichannel cochlear implant contains a number of electrode contacts arranged along its electrode array which is inserted inside the cochlea. These electrode contacts stimulate different locations inside the cochlea to achieve a frequency-based pitch perception which helps in speech understanding. Once the patient is implanted, the audiologists start programming the device to achieve the best hearing outcome. Cochlear implant programming includes allocating specific frequencies to each electrode contact. And since the cochlear implant is aiming to replace the normal cochlear sensation, the frequency allocations are programmed in a way to simulate the exponential logarithmic function of the normal cochlea's frequency map. To have a better understanding of the concepts behind anatomy-based programming, we need to understand the relevant cochlear anatomy and physiology of pitch perception which will be discussed in this chapter. Reaching a patient-specific anatomy-based programming then includes clinical application of measuring the relevant anatomical variables that is not an easy task to perform, and we will discuss the difficulties in this process in this chapter.

2. Relevant cochlear anatomy

The cochlea is a hollow spiral structure in the inner ear that is responsible for the hearing sensation. It is contained within the petrous portion of the temporal bone. The spiral hallow of the cochlea turns around a central bony pyramid called modiolus. A thin bony plate, called the osseous spiral lamina, is connected to the modiolus and divides the bony cochlea incompletely. The cochlear lumen is divided into three spaces by two membranes that are attached to the spiral lamina; the basilar membrane that separates the scala tympani from the scala media and the Reissner's membrane that separates the scala media from the scala vestibuli. The organ of corti is supported on the basilar membrane and contains the hearing sensory cells. From the basilar membrane, nerve fibers travel to the spiral ganglion, a structure that is located closer to the cochlear spiral's axis of rotation and includes neuron cell bodies.

During cochlear implantation, an electrode array is placed in the scala tympani of the cochlea to stimulate the cochlear nerve and induce action potentials. It is still undetermined where these APs are evoked along the sensorineural pathway of the hearing (**Figure 1**) [1].

2.1 Basilar membrane

The acoustic stimulus causes the vibration of the tympanic membrane and in turn the ossicular chain, ending in the vibration of the footplate of the stapes that causes a wave in the perilymphatic fluid inside the scala vestibuli which is transferred to the basilar membrane. Von Bekesy in his Nobel Lecture, in the 1960s, was the first to introduce the

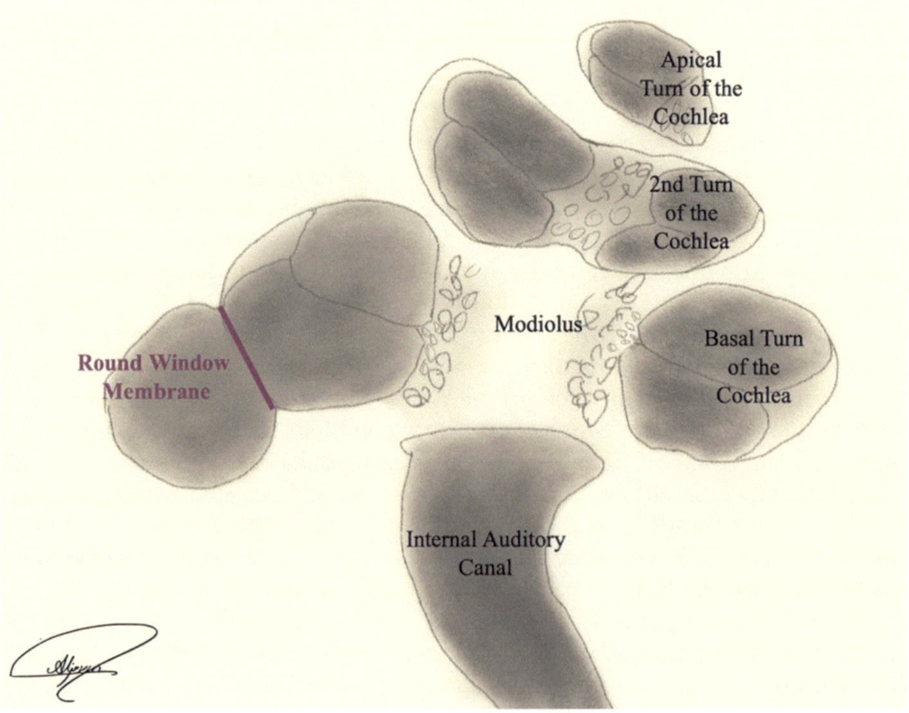

Figure 1.
Showing the anatomy of the cochlea as seen in a mid-modiolar view in a micro-CT image of the temporal bone.

concept of this cochlear traveling wave along the basilar membrane. The maximum vibration amplitude of this wave along the basilar membrane is located in a different place according to the stimulus frequency, resulting in an increased sensitivity of that place in the basilar membrane to that special frequency. The frequency to which the basilar membrane shows the most sensitivity is called the characteristic frequency [2–4].

The physical properties of the basilar membrane and the cochlear fluids determine the characteristic frequencies along the basilar membrane. Although the cochlear structure maintains relatively the same along the length of the cochlea, there are three changes to its physical properties. First, the cochlear lumen decreases from the base toward the apex. Second, the basilar membrane mass is higher in the base in compared to the apex due to the increased number and size of the supporting cells. Third, the basilar membrane is stiffer by about 100-fold at the base in compared to the apex. These changes in the physical properties of the basilar membrane result in a change of the amplitude of the cochlear traveling wave. The wave increases in amplitude while traveling from the base toward the apex, till it reaches the place of the maximum amplitude, beyond which it declines. The place of the maximum amplitude is dependent on the characteristic frequency for that place resulting in a spatial cochlear frequency map. This spatial frequency sensitivity map is what is referred to as the cochlear tonotopicity (**Figure 2**) [5].

The characteristic frequency of each place on the cochlea can be calculated using an equation introduced by Greenwood. In this equation, the input is the vibratory length of the basilar membrane containing the sensory organ of corti [6].

The standard of preoperative evaluation of cochlear implant patients have been either computed tomography (CT), magnetic resonance imaging (MRI), or both for decades now. However, both these imaging techniques lack the spatial resolution needed to visualize the basilar membrane which is needed for the Greenwood frequency eq. [7].

Since the actual measurement of the length of the organ of corti is not feasible during the routine imaging, an estimate is made through a number of steps. The organ of corti on the basilar membrane runs closer to the lateral bony wall of the cochlea.

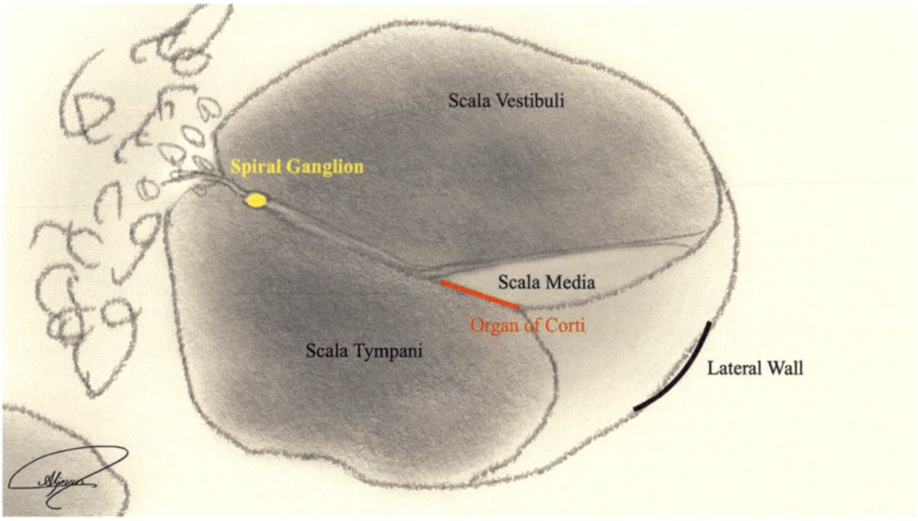

Figure 2.
Illustrating the location of the spiral ganglion, the organ of corti, and the lateral wall as would be seen in a micro-CT image.

Although the lateral bony wall of the cochlea does not contain any special hearing structures, it is of utmost clinical importance. This is because it is easily observed via the routinely performed CT imaging studies that are performed for the evaluation of cochlear implantation patients. Hence, its length has been used as an estimate to the length of the basilar membrane.

2.2 Helicotrema

The helicotrema is the most apical part of the cochlea that lacks basilar membrane. It starts where the scala tympani and the scala vestibuli merge, to the apical end of the cochlear bony wall [8, 9].

An accurate measurement of the basilar membrane length is a prerequisite for anatomy-based programming calculations. The lack of visible boundaries in the end point of the cochlear apex using routine high-resolution CT resulted in an inaccurate estimation of the length of the basilar membrane. Furthermore, the total cochlear rotation is highly variable in the apex, resulting in an additional inaccuracy in the cochlear duct length (CDL) measurement modeling techniques [10–12].

Using synchrotron radiation phase-contrast imaging, the length of the basilar membrane has been found to be highly correlated to the bony cochlear duct length using the following equation:

$$\text{Basilar membrane length} = 0.88(\text{CDL}_{\text{TIP}}) + 3.71. \quad (1)$$

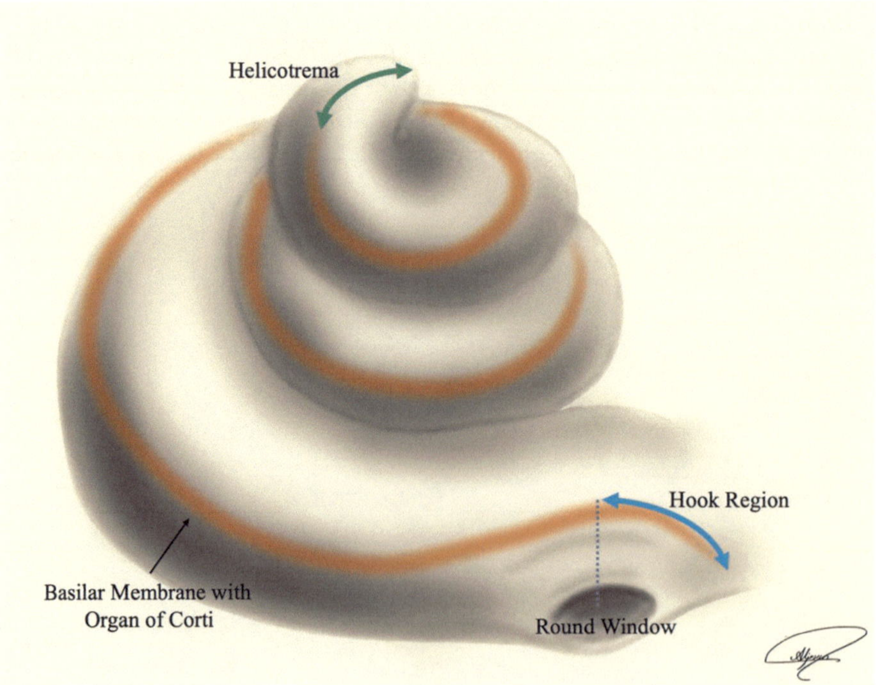

Figure 3.
Illustrating the location of the hook region and the helicotrema in the cochlea. The hook region is the part of the basilar membrane starting before the midpoint of the round window which is the anatomical part that is easily seen in a high-resolution CT. The helicotrema is the part of the cochlear length that lacks basilar membrane structure.

where CDL_{TIP} refers to the length of CDL to the tip of the bony wall of the cochlea.

The use of this correction can help in a more accurate measurement of the basilar membrane [13].

2.3 Hook region

The hook region is the most basal part of the cochlear bony canal, which forms a curvature beyond the level of the round window [14, 15].

The basilar membrane continues in the hook region of the cochlea. This means that for a more accurate calculation of the place-related tonotopic representation, the length of the hook region needs to be considered and corrected. Furthermore, the connective dendrites in the hook region follow a nonradial trajectory from the basilar membrane to the spiral ganglion, which needs to be considered in evaluating the spiral ganglion tonotopic map.

Using synchrotron radiation phase-contrast imaging, an addition of a 2.5 mm as an average of the hook region length can improve the accuracy of the basilar membrane measurement (**Figure 3**) [16].

3. Mechanisms of hearing

3.1 Pitch perception

The pitch of a sound is the subjective perception of that sound on a musical scale [17]. The perception of sound pitch is believed to be determined through two functions: the spatial and temporal cues of the sound. The spatial cues of the sounds are elicited by the place where the peak of electrical stimulation is located in the tonotopic map of the cochlea.

The temporal cues are determined by the precise timing of the action potentials at a certain phase within the cycle of the sound tone, resulting in a specific time interval between the action potentials [18]. The temporal cues have been found to be more of importance in the lower frequencies, after which becoming difficult to detect experimentally, in a phenomenon called phase locking. The level of phase locking has been found to be at about 1–2 kHz depending on the species.

The electrical hearing in cochlear implanted recipients would result in a better synchronization compared to the acoustic hearing, which might suggest a more reliable pitch perception with temporal cues [19, 20].

However, in cochlear implant recipients, 300 Hz was found to be the upper boundary of temporal cue function in pitch perception. It needs to be mentioned that the inability to discriminate temporal cues does not necessarily mean that the temporal information is not processed, as the physiological psychophysiacl studies shown detection of temporal fluctuations as high as 4 kHz [21–23]. This upper limit can affect the ability of CI recipients to recognize melodies and musical intervals and their ability to detect minor changes in frequencies using temporal cues which is present in normal hearing cochlea till up to 4–5 kHz [24–26].

The use of functional MRI in more recent studies have been used in a try to shade more light on the understanding of pitch perception in human, specially that the invasive nature of phase lock measurement has prevented its actual measurement in human. This area however yet needs further study since no consensus has been reached on the tonotopic organization of the auditory brain areas [27–31].

4. Calculation of characteristic frequency

4.1 Calculation of characteristic frequency and anatomy-based frequency allocation

There are mainly two widely known methods to calculate the characteristic frequencies, based on the tonotopic map of the two most probable areas where the electrical stimulus first picked up along the sensorineural elements of the cochlea. First is the Greenwood's function that estimates the characteristic frequencies along the organ of corti. The second is the Stakhovskaya frequency map for the spiral ganglion [32].

Greeenwood equation is a near-logarithmic function relating the frequency to the relative position of the area being studied within the whole length of the organ of corti. The equation is as follows:

$$f = 165.4\left(10^{2.1x} - 0.88\right) \tag{2}$$

where f is the characteristic frequency of the area of interest and x is fractional length of the area or interest along the OC:

$$x = [CDL_{oc} - CDL_{oc}(\theta)]/CDL_{oc} \tag{3}$$

Measuring the length of the organ of corti, which is needed for the Greenwood equation, is still a matter of study. To estimate this length for a CI recipient, a CT image is usually used. The CT image can show the bony boundaries of the cochlea. The use of CT image for this estimation results in a number of inaccuracies. First, the OC is not exactly located in the lateral bony wall, but rather more medially. To overcome this inaccuracy, Alexiades has proposed an equation to correct for the medial position of the OC in relation to the lateral cochlear bony wall as follows:

$$CDL_{oc} = \left[1.71^* \left[1^* 1 : 18^* (A_{oc}) + 2 : 69^* (B_{oc}) - \sqrt{0.72^* A_{oc}{}^* B_{oc}}\right)\right] * 0 : 18 \tag{4}$$

where value A_{oc} is corrected length of the OC for the linear measurement from the round window to the furthest lateral wall on the opposite side of the basal turn of the cochlea, and value B_{oc} is corrected length of the OC for the linear measurement perpendicular to the cochlear opposite lateral walls' diameter.

The second inaccuracy is due to the fact that the cochlear parameters used to measure the CDL use the visible anatomy of the midpoint of the round window as the start point for measurement. This start point disregards the presence of the OC in the hook region, beyond the round window. Recent sychotron imaging-based anatomical studies suggest adding a correction factor of 2.5 mm to the OC length as the mean of hook region length [16]. Although there is a variability in the cochlear height, the effect of this variability on the CDL is still poorly studied, which can be another source of inaccurate CDL estimation [33–35].

Stakhovskaya map, which is the second method to calculate the characteristic frequencies, was driven from the radial trajectory of the organ of corti Greenwood map. This map suggests a constant frequency map according to the angle of the place in the cochlea to be studied with disregard to the anatomical variations in the CDL, OC, and SG lengths. In forming of Stakhovskaya map, two-dimensional cochlear views were used that might not perfectly represent the three-dimensional reality of the cochlea. Furthermore, the relation of the OC and SG does not continue as perfect radial trajectories since the length of the OC continues beyond the level where the SG

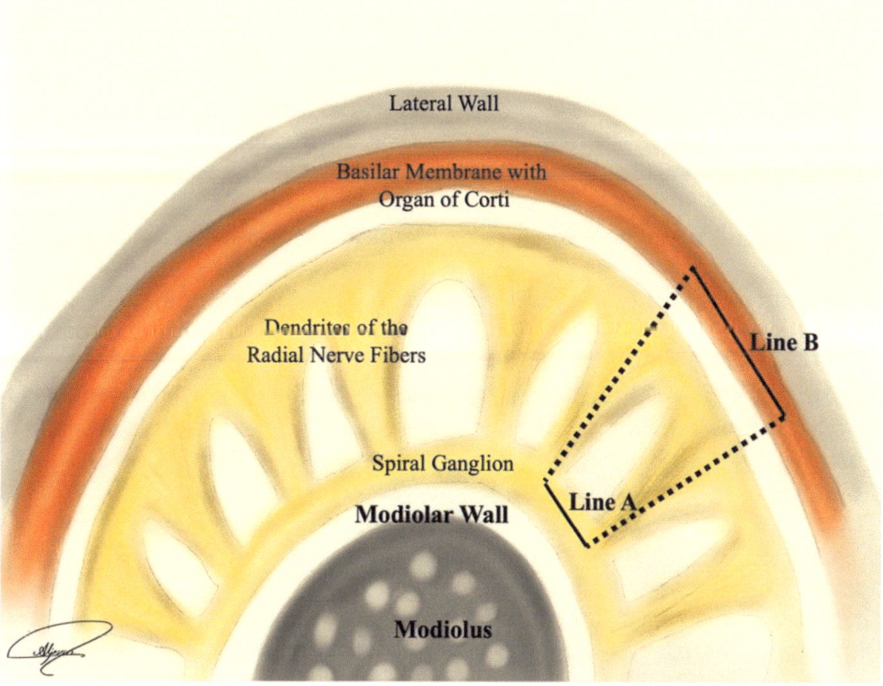

Figure 4.
Stakhovskaya calculated the spiral ganglion tonotopicity map as a function of basilar membrane tonotopicity map, by correlating the length of line A, representing the spiral ganglion length, in relation to line B, representing the basilar membrane length.

length ends, making the more apical areas of the SG highly condensed with OC representing dendrites (**Figure 4**).

Using the 3D synchrotron radiation phase-contrast imaging, the spiral ganglion angle-frequency function can be calculated using the following equation:

$$f = 2^{(-0.12\theta+160/12)} \tag{5}$$

where θ stands for the angular depth, measured from the center of the RW.

These measures were not observed to significantly differ from that of Stakhovskaya frequency map [36]. The spiral ganglion tonotopicity is highly compacted at its apex, which makes it extremely difficult to selectively excite low-frequency neurons.

4.2 Calculation of the frequency-to-place mismatch

The amount of the frequency-to-place mismatch is calculated by determining the difference in the frequency presented by each electrode contact and the characteristic frequency of the place where this electrode contact is located.

4.3 Determinants of frequency-to-place mismatch

Frequency-to-place mismatch happens when the electrode presents a frequency stimulus to a place in the cochlea that does not match the frequency to which that place shows the highest sensitivity to.

This discrepancy is due to the relative misplacement of two places with same frequency to each other, namely the place of the electrode contact that is programmed to stimulate a specific frequency and the place in the cochlea with that same characteristic frequency.

After surgical placing of the electrode contact, the place of the electrode contact is determined and to match the frequency-to-place, the fitting of the electrode contact can be changed to adjust to the characteristic frequency of the cochlea where the contact is located.

Using a default frequency map for all patients has shown to result in a significant mismatch.

The first determinant of the mismatch is the length of the electrode. The current electrode designs have different active stimulating ranges in which the contacts are located. The Greenwood equation takes into consideration the location of the electrode contacts to calculate the characteristic frequency of that place. Given the same default map for all designs, the different lengths of the electrode arrays result in different insertion depth with full insertion, and therefore in different characteristic frequencies they face, which in turn results in different extent of mismatch (**Figure 5**) [37].

The second determinant of the mismatch is the cochlear duct length, which is the other variable in the Greenwood equation. There is a vast variability in the cochlear duct length in normal population that ranges from 19.71 to 45.6 mm. To add more to this complexity, there are a large number of cochlear implant recipients who have cochlear anomalies that can affect the cochlear duct length (**Figure 6**) [32, 35, 38, 39].

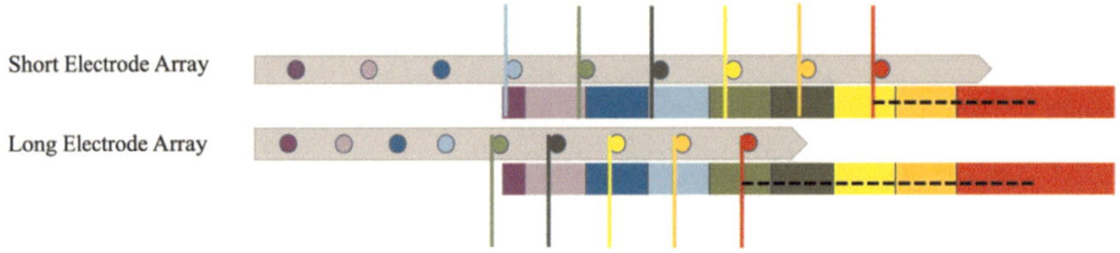

Figure 5.
The effect of the electrode length on the magnitude of the mismatch, illustrated as dashed black line, when default frequency mapping is used.

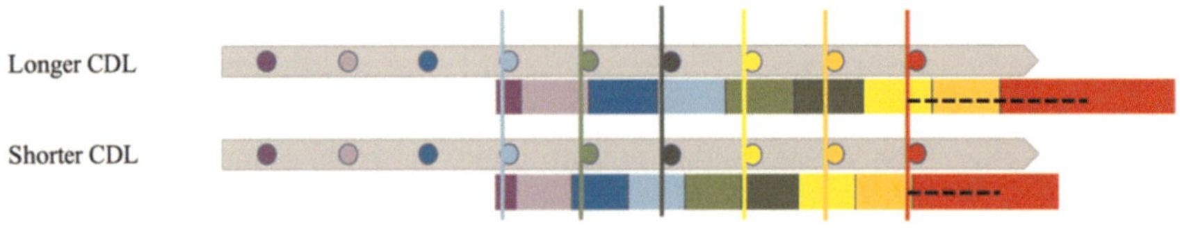

Figure 6.
The effect of the cochlear duct length (CDL) on the magnitude of the mismatch, illustrated as dashed black line, when default frequency mapping is used.

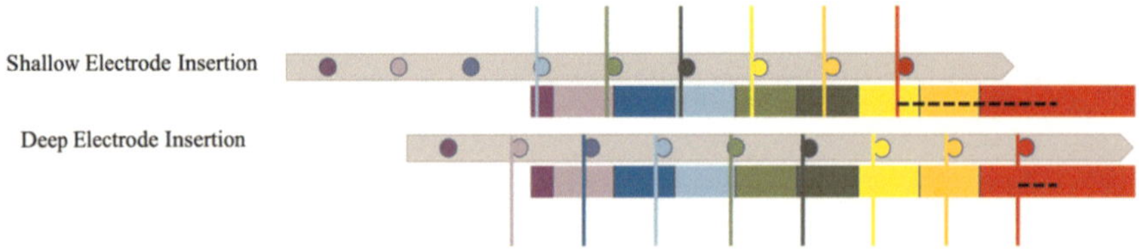

Figure 7.
The effect of the degree of insertion on the magnitude of the mismatch, illustrated as dashed black line, when default frequency mapping is used.

The last determinant is the surgical position of the electrode array according to the depth of insertion (**Figure 7**).

5. The importance of frequency-to-place mismatch

As discussed in the previous section, the impact of frequency-to-place mismatch is still under study. However, theoretically there are special scenarios where the frequency-to-place mismatch is theorized to be of more importance.

One of them is in the patients who have any sort of hearing memory, where they have had acoustic hearing that was lost afterward. This category includes a large portion of implanted patients with various etiologies that can either be a progressive hearing loss, presbycusis, sudden sensorineural hearing loss or patients who lost their hearing after temporal bone trauma or ontological surgery. It is assumed that these patients would remember the characteristic frequency of each location in their cochlea and would compare the electric hearing to their memory of the acoustic hearing.

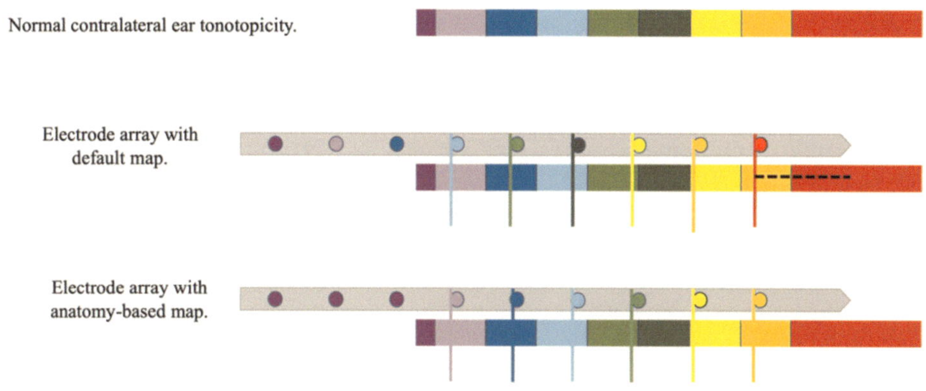

Figure 8.
The difference between default and anatomy-based map in a case of single sided deafness.

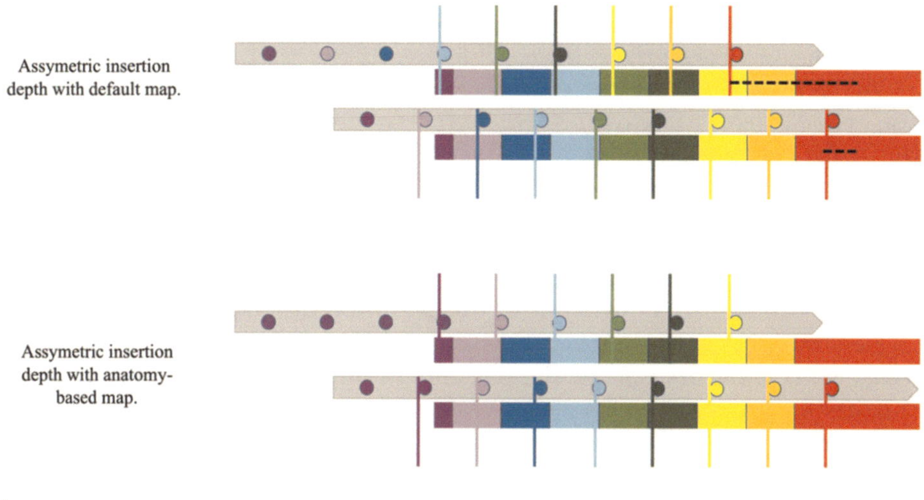

Figure 9.
The difference between default and anatomy-based map in a case with asymmetrical insertion depth.

Anatomy-based programming was found to be associated with a better auditory outcome in postlingual adults [40].

The second category are patients with single-sided hearing, even if they do not have any hearing memory in the deafened ear, and these patients could compare the hearing in the implanted ear to the hearing in the contralateral normal ear with the normal tonotopicity. And it has been shown that patients with single sided deafness (SSD) have a high rate of nonuse and not all will cope to the use of CI (**Figure 8**).

The third category are patients with bilateral CI who have different insertion depth, different electrode lengths, or different cochlear duct length in the two cochleae. Giving an anatomy-based fitting to these patients would result in a more balanced and symmetrical hearing and is theorized to have a more acceptable presentation to the brain (**Figure 9**).

6. The clinical impact of frequency-to-place mismatch

Considering the three determinants of the frequency-to-place mismatch, the effect of each of these determinants on the auditory and speech outcomes can be considered as an indirect effect of a better frequency-to-place matching.

Numerous articles have shown a better outcome with longer electrodes and deeper insertion including speech recognition scores. The studies also showed that these superior auditory outcomes appear in the early post-activation period and were sustained in long-term use [41–48]. Patients with single-sided deafness showed improved head shadow benefits as well as better spatial release of masking with a better frequency-to-place matching [49]. Better auditory outcomes have been found in association with a better frequency-to-place matching in elderly adults, which may be of particular benefit to them considering the age-related deficit in the auditory processing [40].

7. Areas to explore

There is still unclear where the site of stimulation is in the cochlea, weather it is the organ of corti, the spiral ganglion, a combination of both, or even somewhere else.

While the organ of corti continues till the level of the helicotrema in the apical turn, the spiral ganglion does not go further than half of the second turn. Argue can be made weather there is a need for a deeper cochlear insertion and longer electrodes to cover all the length of the OC or is it enough that we reach up to the level where the SG ends. And although the OC course and length is more predictable using the routine CT imaging, the SG has an unpredictable and steep and condense tonotopic presentation at its more apical end and would be extremely difficult to achieve a proper frequency-to-place matching at that area (**Figure 10**).

The other consideration for a perfect frequency-to-place matching is the fact that to achieve that, we are losing some of the low-frequency perception that is not covered with the electrode in the OC mapping specially. This area of noncoverage will be more with shorter electrodes. However, it needs to be considered that the normal hearing covers up to 20 Hz as the lower frequency limit, and the effect of covering this low level of frequency with cochlear implant is not supposed to be high in speech perception and intelligibility [50]. Future studies on the site of the first stimulus generation are needed to shade light on this matter (**Figure 11**).

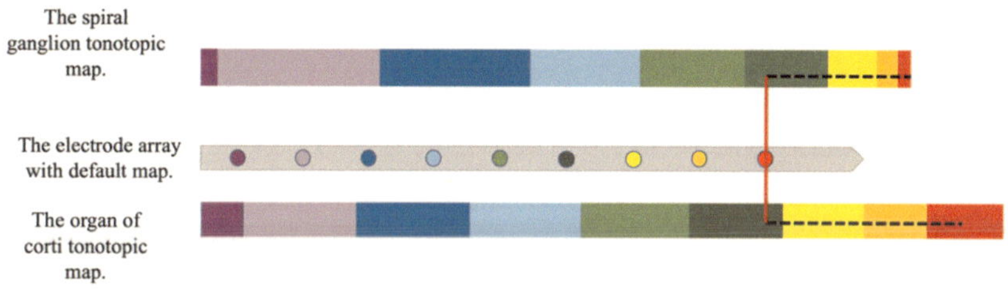

Figure 10.
The difference between the frequency-to-place mismatch using the organ of corti map in compared to the spiral ganglion map.

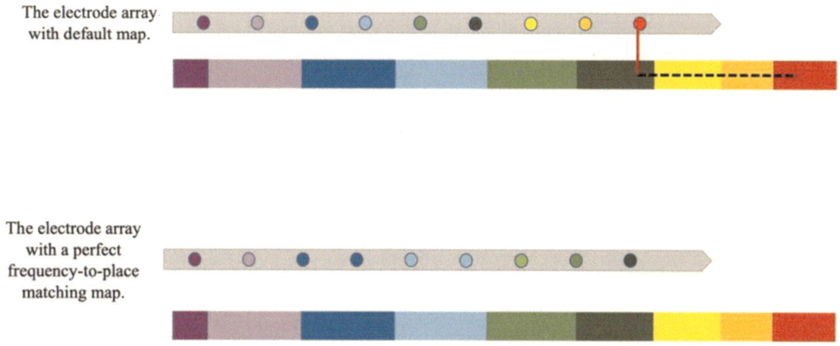

Figure 11.
The difference between default and a perfect anatomy-based map in the ability to cover the lower frequencies.

8. Conclusion

A default frequency fitting results in a wide variability of frequency-to-place mismatch. The variability of the magnitude of the frequency-to-place mismatch is dependent on the degree of insertion, length of the electrode, and the cochlear duct length. The anatomy-based fitting provides a personalized frequency map for the CI users that aim to better imitate the tonotopocity of the normal cochlea. The current evidence suggests that anatomy-based fitting can enhance the CI user benefit.

Conflict of interest

"The author declares no conflict of interest."

Author details

Isra Aljazeeri[1,2*], Yassin Abdelsamad[3] and Abdulrahman Hagr[2]

1 Aljaber Ophthalmology and Otolaryngology Hospital, Otolaryngology Department, Ministry of Health, Ahsa, Saudi Arabia

2 King Abdullah Ear Specialist Center (KAESC), College of Medicine, King Saud University Medical City (KSUMC), King Saud University, Riyadh, Saudi Arabia

3 Research Department, MED-EL GmbH, Riyadh, Saudi Arabia

*Address all correspondence to: isra.aljazeeri@gmail.com

References

[1] Clark WW, Ohlemiller KK. Anatomy and Physiology of Hearing for Audiologists. New York: Thomson Delmar Learning, Singular; 2008

[2] Olson ES, Duifhuis H, Steele CR. Von Békésy and cochlear mechanics. Hearing Research. 2012;**293**(1–2):31-43

[3] Manley GA, Narins PM, Fay RR. Experiments in comparative hearing: Georg von Békésy and beyond. Hearing Research. 2012;**293**(1–2):44-50

[4] Békésy G. Concerning the pleasures of observing, and the mechanics of the inner ear. Nobel Lect 1961

[5] Kim J, Koo M. Mass and stiffness impact on the middle ear and the cochlear partition. Journal of Audiology and Otology. 2015;**19**(12):1-6. Available from: https://www.ncbi.nlm.nih.gov/pmc/articles/PMC4491943/pdf/jao-19-1.pdf

[6] Greenwood DD. A cochlear frequency-position function for several species–29 years later. The Journal of the Acoustical Society of America. 2021; **87**(6):2592-2605. Available from: https://pubmed.ncbi.nlm.nih.gov/2373794/

[7] Elfarnawany M, Alam SR, Rohani SA, Zhu N, Agrawal SK, Ladak HM. Micro-CT versus synchrotron radiation phase contrast imaging of human cochlea. Journal of Microscopy. 2016;**265**(3):349-357

[8] Braun K, Böhnke F, Stark T. Three-dimensional representation of the human cochlea using micro-computed tomography data: Presenting an anatomical model for further numerical calculations. Acta Oto-Laryngologica. 2012;**132**(6):603-613

[9] Hilding AC. Studies on the Otic labyrinth. Annals of Otology, Rhinology & Laryngology. 1955;**64**(1):278-290

[10] Alexiades G, Dhanasingh A, Jolly C. Method to estimate the complete and two-turn Cochlear duct length. Otology & Neurotology. 2015;**36**(5):904-907

[11] Erixon E, Rask-Andersen H. How to predict cochlear length before cochlear implantation surgery. Acta Oto-Laryngologica. 2013;**133**(12):1258-1265

[12] Koch RW, Elfarnawany M, Zhu N, Ladak HM, Agrawal SK. Evaluation of Cochlear duct length computations using synchrotron radiation phase-contrast imaging. Otology & Neurotology. 2017; **38**(6):e92-e99

[13] Helpard L, Li H, Rask-Andersen H, Ladak HM, Agrawal SK. Characterization of the human helicotrema: implications for cochlear duct length and frequency mapping. Journal of Otolaryngology - Head & Neck Surgery. 2020;**49**:6

[14] Li PMMC, Wang H, Northrop C, Merchant SN, Nadol JB. Anatomy of the round window and hook region of the cochlea with implications for Cochlear implantation and other Endocochlear surgical procedures. Otology & Neurotology. 2007;**28**(5):641-648

[15] Stidham KR, Rober JB. Cochlear hook anatomy: Evaluation of the spatial relationship of the basal Cochlear duct to middle ear landmarks. Acta Oto-Laryngologica. 1999;**119**(7):773-777

[16] Helpard L, Li H, Rohani SA, Rask-Andersen H, Ladak HM, Agrawal S. Three-dimensional modeling and measurement of the human Cochlear hook region: Considerations for tonotopic mapping. Otology & Neurotology. 2021;**42**(6):e658-e665

[17] JHE C, Gonzalez DL, Piro O. Pitch perception: A dynamical-systems

perspective. Proceedings of the National Academy of Sciences. 2001;**98**(9): 4855-4859. Available from: http://www.iact.ugr-csic.es/personal/julyan_cartwright/PDFs/37_2001_PNAS.pdf

[18] Oxenham AJ, Micheyl C, Keebler MV, Loper A, Santurette S. Pitch perception beyond the traditional existence region of pitch. Proceedings of the National Academy of Sciences. 2011; **108**(18):7629-7634. Available from: https://www.pnas.org/content/pnas/108/18/7629.full.pdf

[19] Litvak L, Delgutte B, Eddington D. Auditory nerve fiber responses to electric stimulation: Modulated and unmodulated pulse trains. The Journal of the Acoustical Society of America. 2001; **110**(1):368-379

[20] Dynes SBC, Delgutte B. Phase-locking of auditory-nerve discharges to sinusoidal electric stimulation of the cochlea. Hearing Research. 1992;**58**(1): 79-90

[21] Shannon RV. Temporal modulation transfer functions in patients with cochlear implants. The Journal of the Acoustical Society of America. 1992; **91**(4):2156-2164

[22] Zeng F-G. Temporal pitch in electric hearing. Hearing Research. 2002;**174**(1–2):101-106

[23] Bacon S, Fay RR. Compression: From Cochlea to Cochlear Implants. 2004th Edition. Springer Handbook of Auditory Research, Springer Science & Business Media; 2006

[24] Semal C, Demany L. The upper limit of "musical" pitch. Music Perception. 1990;**8**(2):165-175

[25] Attneave F, Olson RK. Pitch as a medium: A new approach to psychophysical scaling. The American Journal of Psychology. 1971;**84**(2):147

[26] Burns EM, Feth LL. High-freqeuncy pitch perception. The Journal of the Acoustical Society of America. 1983;**73**(S1):S44-S44

[27] Langers DRM, van Dijk P. Mapping the tonotopic Organization in Human Auditory Cortex with minimally salient acoustic stimulation. Cerebral Cortex. 2011;**22**(9):2024-2038

[28] Woods DL, Stecker GC, Rinne T, Herron TJ, Cate AD, Yund EW, et al. Functional maps of human auditory cortex: Effects of acoustic features and attention. PLoS ONE. 2009;**4**(4):e5183

[29] Talavage TM, Sereno MI, Melcher JR, Ledden PJ, Rosen BR, Dale AM. Tonotopic organization in human auditory cortex revealed by progressions of frequency sensitivity. Journal of Neurophysiology. 2004;**91**(3): 1282-1296

[30] Da Costa S, van der Zwaag W, Marques JP, Frackowiak RSJ, Clarke S, Saenz M. Human primary auditory cortex follows the shape of Heschl's gyrus. Journal of Neuroscience. 2011; **31**(40):14067-14075

[31] Griffiths TD, Hall DA. Mapping pitch representation in neural ensembles with fMRI. The Journal of Neuroscience. 2012;**32**(39):13343-13347. Available from: https://www.ncbi.nlm.nih.gov/pmc/articles/PMC6621372/

[32] Stakhovskaya O, Sridhar D, Bonham BH, Leake PA. Frequency map for the human Cochlear spiral ganglion: Implications for Cochlear implants. Journal of the Association for Research in Otolaryngology. 2007;**8**(2):220-233

[33] Zahara D, Dewi RD, Aboet A, Putranto FM, Lubis ND, Ashar T.

Variations in Cochlear size of Cochlear implant candidates. International Archives of Otorhinolaryngology. 2018; **23**(02):184-190

[34] Alshalan A, Abdelsamad Y, Assiri M, Alsanosi A. Cochlear implantation: The variation in Cochlear height. Ear, Nose & Throat Journal. 2022;**17**:0145

[35] Khurayzi T, Almuhawas F, Sanosi A. Direct measurement of cochlear parameters for automatic calculation of the cochlear duct length. Annals of Saudi Medicine. 2020;**40**(3):212-218

[36] Helpard L, Li H, Rohani SA, Zhu N, Rask-Andersen H, Agrawal S, et al. An approach for individualized Cochlear frequency mapping determined from 3D synchrotron radiation phase-contrast imaging. IEEE Transactions on Biomedical Engineering. 2021;**68**(12): 3602-3611

[37] Dhanasingh A, Jolly C. An overview of cochlear implant electrode array designs. Hearing Research. 2017;**356**: 93-103

[38] Grover M, Sharma S, Singh SN, Kataria T, Lakhawat RS, Sharma MP. Measuring cochlear duct length in Asian population: Worth giving a thought! European Archives of Oto-Rhino-Laryngology. 2018;**275**(3):725-728

[39] Alanazi A, Alzhrani F. Comparison of cochlear duct length between the Saudi and non-Saudi populations. Annals of Saudi Medicine. 2018;**38**(2):125-129

[40] Canfarotta MW, O'Connell BP, Buss E, Pillsbury HC, Brown KD, Dillon MT. Influence of age at Cochlear implantation and frequency-to-place mismatch on early speech recognition in adults. Otolaryngology–Head and Neck Surgery. 2020;**162**(6):926-932

[41] Canfarotta MW, Dillon MT, Brown KD, Pillsbury HC, Dedmon MM, O'Connell BP. Insertion depth and Cochlear implant speech recognition outcomes: A comparative study of 28- and 31.5-mm Lateral Wall arrays. Otology & Neurotology. 2021;**43**(2): 183-189

[42] Boyd PJ. Potential benefits from deeply inserted Cochlear implant electrodes. Ear and Hearing. 2011;**32**(4): 411-427

[43] Hamzavi J, Arnoldner C. Effect of deep insertion of the cochlear implant electrode array on pitch estimation and speech perception. Acta Oto-Laryngologica. 2006;**25**:1-1

[44] Lee F-P, Hsu H-T, Lin Y-S, Hung S-C. Effects of the electrode location on tonal discrimination and speech perception of mandarin-speaking patients with a cochlear implant. The Laryngoscope. 2012;**122**(6):1366-1378

[45] Gani M, Valentini G, Sigrist A, Kós M-I, Boëx C. Implications of deep electrode insertion on Cochlear implant fitting. Journal of the Association for Research in Otolaryngology. 2007;**8**(1): 69-83

[46] van Besouw RM, Forrester L, Crowe ND, Rowan D. Simulating the effect of interaural mismatch in the insertion depth of bilateral cochlear implants on speech perception. The Journal of the Acoustical Society of America. 2013;**134**(2):1348-1357

[47] Buchman CA, Dillon MT, King ER, Adunka MC, Adunka OF, Pillsbury HC. Influence of Cochlear implant insertion depth on performance. Otology & Neurotology. 2014;**35**(10):1773-1779

[48] Canfarotta MW, Dillon MT, Buchman CA, Buss E, O'Connell BP,

Rooth MA, et al. Long-term influence of electrode Array length on speech recognition in Cochlear implant users. The Laryngoscope. 2020;**131**(4):892-897

[49] Zhou X, Li H, Galvin JJ, Fu Q-J, Yuan W. Effects of insertion depth on spatial speech perception in noise for simulations of cochlear implants and single-sided deafness. International Journal of Audiology. 2016;**56**(sup2): S41-S48

[50] Dincer D'Alessandro H, Ballantyne D, Boyle PJ, De Seta E, DeVincentiis M, Mancini P. Temporal fine structure processing, pitch, and speech perception in adult Cochlear implant recipients. Ear and Hearing. 2018;**39**(4):679-686

Chapter 6

Perceptual Learning of Uncategorized Arabic Phonemes among Congenitally Deaf, Non-native Children with Cochlear Implants

Farheen Naz Anis and Cila Umat

Abstract

The advancement in cochlear implant (CI) technologies and how CIs help their users have far exceeded expectations. Speech perception remains the focus of many studies related to cochlear implant clinical research to ensure the technology maximizes the benefits to be obtained by CI users. This chapter will discuss the perception of non-native sounds among congenitally deaf pediatric CI users, specifically emphasizing Arabic consonants. This language is used and learned by billions of non-native Arabs worldwide. Non-native auditory signals are perceived differently by children with CI due to speech processor signal processing and native language learning effects. This study measured the perceptual learning of uncategorized-dispersed-assimilated Arabic consonants for a group of non-native children with CI using a newly developed, *FizBil*© bottom-up, customized software training module. The framework and hypothetical pathway will be discussed.

Keywords: cochlear implants, children, uncategorized non-native arabic phonemes, perceptual learning, bottom-up training

1. Introduction

Superior speech perception is perhaps the most significant outcome of cochlear implantation and directly correlates with linguistic, social, and learning outcomes [1–4]. Consequently, children who can function well auditorily with a cochlear implant (CI) can attend mainstream schools [1, 5–7] and learn a new language [8–13] within the normative range [14–17]. Furthermore, research shows that children with CI perform well on non-native perceptual listening tasks [11, 18–22]. Conversely, there is evidence showing that normal hearing [23] and deaf children with CI struggle with non-native phonemes perception [6, 7], production [24], and language learning [12, 25, 26].

Speech sound is a complex signal that carries information in the form of acoustic cues. These acoustic cues (usually in combination) represent the phonological categories, that is, place of articulation, manner of articulation, and voicing. To recognize the speech sounds, listeners need to categorize these acoustic signals. Hearing with a cochlear implant is not analogous to acoustic hearing. The auditory brain of children with CI processes signals differently from their normal-hearing (NH) peers. In CI, input signals are coded by electrical pulses, while the brain processes acoustic input signals in normal-hearing listeners. Complex temporal and spatial excitation patterns represent a sound signal in approximately 20,000 auditory neurons [27] in a typical auditory pathway. On the other hand, currently, available electrodes for commercial CI systems have a maximum of 22 excitation points for neurons to deliver sound signals to the auditory brain. A comparison of signal pathways for sound processing *via* acoustic hearing and a cochlear implant is shown in **Figure 1**.

Therefore, children with CI need to learn speech perception from the poorer frequency resolution than their NH peers [28–30]. Apart from a poorer frequency resolution, cross-channel interactions [30], electrode discrimination ability, and

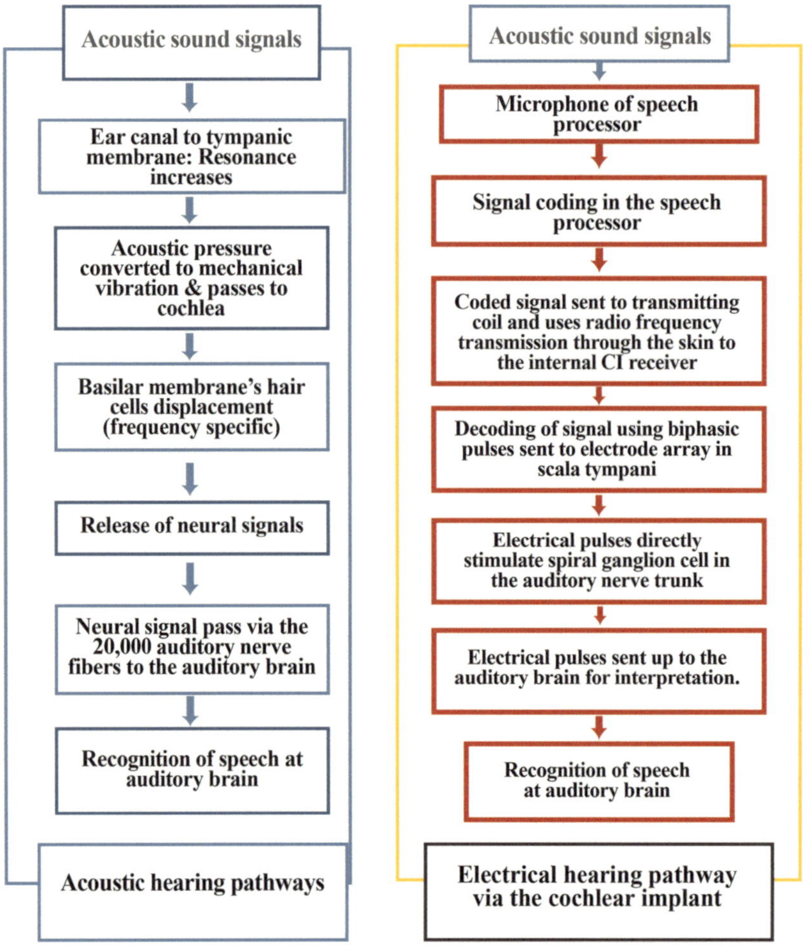

Figure 1.
Comparison of signal pathways for sound processing via *normal acoustic hearing and electrical hearing via a cochlear implant.*

place-pitch shifting due to electrode insertion position [28, 29, 31] are some other factors contributing in poorer speech perception scores in children with CI as compared to their NH peers. Phoneme perception is a categorical process that involves the classification and grouping of the information-bearing acoustic signal. Phonological features information is conveyed *via* multiple cues. For example, the features of voice and manner are transmitted *via* the temporal cues, namely: the envelope and the periodic cues. On the other hand, the temporal fine structures and spectral-domain, that is, transition, coded the place of articulation [30–32]. Research showed that phonemes perception scores for children with CI were generally poorer than the NH children matched for their hearing age. The hearing deprivation period may play an important role [32] in poorer native language speech perception performance. Non-native children with CI learn to produce and maintain the voicing of articulation of native and non-native phonemes [8, 18, 19]. Literature review revealed that CI users show systematic deficits in perceiving phonological features, especially place feature [28, 30, 32] that relies heavily on spectral information. For CI listeners who are less able to accurately discriminate the place of articulation of even native phonemes [30, 32–35], the difficulty level is more pronounced for the non-native phonological features.

Non-Arab Muslims around the globe listen, read, and learn Al-Quran daily to fulfill their religious obligations and prayers. Likewise, children start listening to Al-Quran from a young age when they visit mosques and religious gatherings with their parents. A large body of research indicates that the perception of non-native phonemes is influenced by the native language phonological inventory in normal hearing (NH) [36–43]. In recent years, there has been renewed interest in the non-native perception among CI users [6–22]. Generally, according to the perception assimilation model for non-native languages (PAM-L2), a typical hearing listener's capacity to perceive a non-native phoneme is influenced by the phonological features of their native language [43]. Listeners use native articulatory patterns to detect the similarities of non-native phonemes with their native languages [37–40, 43–46], a process known as *assimilation.* Various possible assimilation categories for non-native phonemes fall within the perceptual space of native language. Malay and Arabic phonological repertoires are generally different [37, 39]. Arabic has unique, distinctive phonological features that do not exist in the Malay phonology repertoire. Therefore, Malay speakers face difficulties recognizing these Arabic sounds from Al-Quran [36, 47]. Evidence shows that posterior and emphatic fricatives ([/q/ ق], [/χ/ خ], [/ʁ/ غ], [/ħ/ ح], [/ʕ/ ع], [/h/ ه], and [/ðˤ/ ظ]) are most difficult sound to utter accurately by NH school-age children [6, 23, 24]. However, in Malaysia, children are exposed to Arabic phonemes in early childhood, that is, 5.0–6.0 years [23, 24]. Consequently, it is anticipated that NH children can develop good perception and recognition skills for Arabic phonemes and acquire reading skills in different writing scripts. **Table 1** compares Arabic & Malay phonological inventory.

Hereafter, it is expected that Malay listeners have a degree of perceptual difficulties with Arabic phonemes as many Malaysians study Arabic as part of the National school curriculum. It is predictable that Arabic language phonological categories fall within the Malay perceptual space due to the frequent use of Arabic in Malay culture. However, our earlier study [6, 7] has shown that for unfamiliar phonemes phonological features' information transmission depends on the category formation in the perceptual space of listeners. It was found that unfamiliar phonemes with a unique category of secondary articulation (/dˤ, ðˤ, sˤ, tˤ/) show dispersed uncategorized assimilation. The unfamiliar phonemes (/q, ħ, ʕ/) with the close phonological

	Bilabial	Labio-dental	Dental	Alveolar	Post-alveolar	Palatal	Velar	Uvular	Pharyngeal	Glottal
Plosive	p **b**			**t d** *tˤ dˤ*			**k**	*q*		ʔ
Nasal	m			n		ɲ	ŋ			
Trill				r						
Fricative		(f)	*θ ð* *ðˤ*	s (z) *sˤ*	(ʃ)		ɣ	*χ*	*ħ ʕ*	h
Affricate				ʤ						
Glides	w				j					
Liquid			l							

IPA symbol to the right represents a voiced phoneme, while the symbol to the left represents a voiceless phoneme.

Key	Black regular	Only occur in Malay inventory
	Blue bold	Occur in both language inventories (familiar for Malay listeners)
	Italic with bracket	Only borrowed words in Malaysian inventory
	Red Italic	Only occur in Arabic inventory (unfamiliar for Malay listeners). These cons

Source: [6, 7, 47].

Table 1.
Comparison of Malay-Arabic phonological inventory.

boundaries with some familiar consonants (/k, h, ʔ) show focalized, uncategorized assimilation. On the other hand, unfamiliar phonemes with a unique subcategory without secondary articulation and close phonological boundaries (/χ, ʁ/) show clustered uncategorized assimilation.

Arabic, the Al-Quran language, is learned by 2.2 billion non-native listeners and readers worldwide. Parents in the non-Arab country send their children to special learning classes for Arabic listening and reading skills. In Malaysia, such as many non-Arabian Muslim countries, Arabic learning is linked with religion and taught in religious schools [23, 24]. On the other hand, parents of children with CI consider Al-Quran education as fundamental for their CI children for their normal-hearing siblings. Therefore, it is essential to understand the Arabic phonemes perception process in children with CI. Therefore, this study was designed to answer whether perceptual learning for unfamiliar non-native phonological features (posterior place or emphatic manner) [6, 7] occurs with customized training. In this study, ***FizBil***©, a software-based, bottom-up training module with specific interstimulus intervals for children with CI was developed, and formative evaluation was done on a small group of NH and CI children. The result of training with the *FizBil*© software from one child with CI who completed the 12-week training program will be reported and discussed.

2. Conceptual framework for design, development, and formative evaluation

The following underlying theories were considered in designing this perceptual training module, which involved identification and discrimination. In addition, a hypothetical pathway shown in **Figure 2** was proposed as the conceptual framework to explain the results of this study. **Figure 2** demonstrates that non-native speech perception depends on categorizing composite sound signals within the auditory brain. Perceptual categorization is based on familiarity. Native phonological features subcategories build up within the listener's perceptual space with signal exposure. According to the signal detection theory (SDT), perceptual categorization of a phoneme is a decision-making process [52, 53]. Perceptual categorization is established on the distance between the perceptual peaks of two signals [54–56]. The identification task [39, 41, 57–60] helps listeners attend to relevant between-category differences *via* top-down processing. In contrast, discrimination tasks [42, 48–51, 57, 61] focus on within-category variability, that is, bottom-up perception [59]. As illustrated in **Figure 2**, children with CI need discrimination training to sharpen the categorization cues [41, 48–51, 60, 61]. Our earlier study [6, 7] revealed more than one phonological feature category mismatch among children with CI. A processing time of 10–500 msec was needed for the discrimination task [49, 62–67].

According to the American Psychological Association [68], *"perceptual learning occurs when repeated exposure enhances the ability to discriminate between two (or more) otherwise confusable stimuli."* Therefore, perceptual learning is the ability to discriminate information from closely related signals with training. Speech perceptual difficulties in non-native listening tasks are well studied and documented [36–45, 69–76]. There are two very well-studied models of speech perception: First, the speech learning model (SLM)

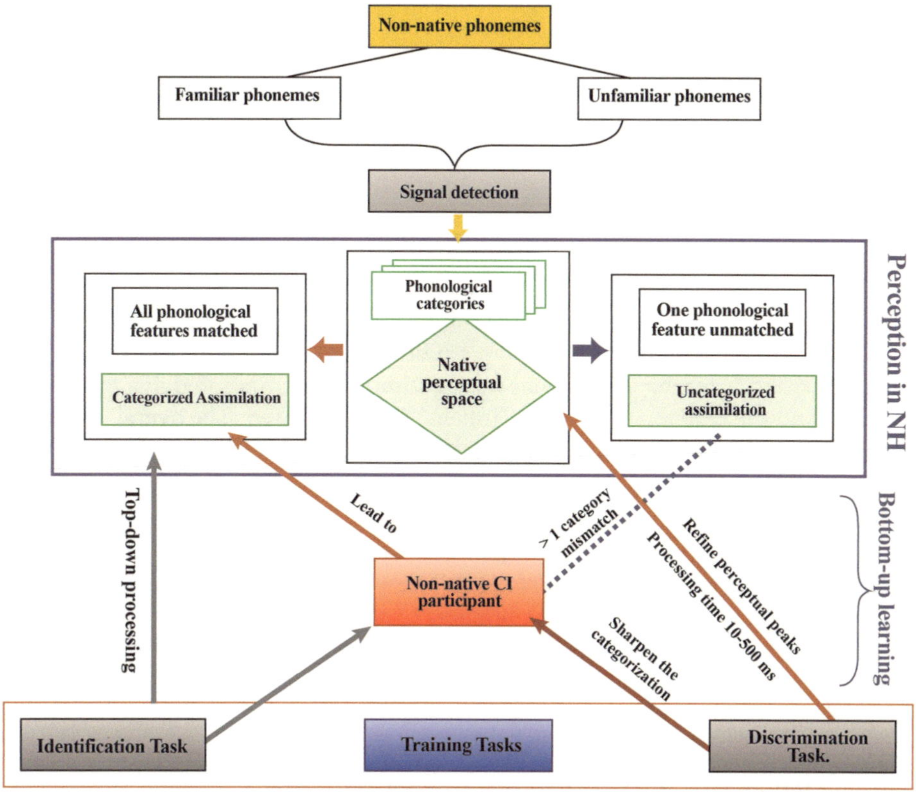

Figure 2.
The conceptualized pathway of signal detection and assimilation of non-native phonemes involves top-down and bottom-up signal processing. Source: [29, 31, 35, 48–51].

suggests a strong positive correlation between the perception of non-native sounds and their production accuracies [70, 71]. Secondly, the perceptual assimilation model (PAM) further elaborates that non-native speech perception difficulties are related to the phonological or acoustic feature perception [36, 38–40, 45, 69] and disembarked from the maturation of native language perceptual space [37, 43, 44]. Hence, improving perception could improve non-native phonemes production [36–44, 70–72, 75].

2.1 Study objectives

The specific objectives of this study were to design (Phase I) and develop (Phase II), to conduct formative evaluation (Phase III) of software-based and perceptual learning (Phase IV) of Arabic phonemes for Malay children with CI utilizing discrimination and identification tasks. Specifically, the following were the objectives:

a. To determine the specific interstimulus interval (ISI) needed by children with CI for speech discrimination tasks.

b. To evaluate the program code for the software ***FizBil***©.

c. To examine the suitability of the graphical user interface for NH children.

d. To scrutinize the suitability of the graphical user interface for children with CI.

e. To examine whether the customized bottom-up training using identification and discrimination tasks improved the perceptual learning index (d' score).

3. Methodology

3.1 Research design

This research was a design, development, and training experiment. The study consists of four phases in which four pilot studies and one case study were carried out. Each study was a listening experiment where stimuli were presented in a controlled condition, and the listener's responses (tokens) were collected. The overall methodological design and summary of all the pilot studies are shown in **Table 2**.

3.2 Research location

Pilot studies A and D, which involved children with CI, were conducted in the soundproof audiology rooms in the Audiology Clinic, Universiti Kebangsaan Malaysia (UKM), Jalan Temerloh, Kuala Lumpur. Pilot studies B and C, which involved NH children, were conducted at the participants' homes with test items presented *via* the loudspeaker on the laptop.

3.3 Demographic characteristics of research participants

The research participants in this study comprised of two groups: (i) The test group (CI children) and (ii) the control group (NH children)

Phase	Exp	Native	Hearing	N	Purpose	Experimental condition	Tokens
I	Pilot A	Malay	CI	2	To determine the suitable inter-stimulus interval (ISI) for CI children training	12 stimuli × 3 ph. pairs × 3track × 4RT = 432 tokens (4 conditions (ds)) (1 condition (id))	3456
II	Pilot B	Arab	NH	2	To check the program code	30 stimuli × 4 phonemes × 3 contrast × 2 tasks = 720 token	1440 + 720
	Pilot C	Malay	NH	5	To check the suitability of the user interface for children	30 stimuli × 1 phoneme × 3 contrasts × 2 tasks = 180 tokens	900
III	Pilot D	Malay	CI	2	To examine the suitability of the user interface for CI children	30 stimuli × 4 phonemes × 3 contrasts × 2 task (2 conditions)	1440
IV	Training case study	Malay	CI	1	To examine the customized bottom-up training using identification and discrimination tasks improved the perceptual learning index (d' score).	30 stimuli × 4 phonemes × 3 contrasts × 2 task (Pretest)	720
						30 stimuli × 4 phonemes × 3 contrasts × 2 Task × 4 training with feedback	2880
						30 stimuli × 4 phonemes × 3 contrasts × 2 task (posttest)	720

Table 2.
Overview of methodological research design for the study.

3.3.1 Test Group (CI: Pilot studies A, D, and training study)

A total of five Malay deaf children with CI were recruited for the study from the UKM Cochlear Implant Program. Two children participated in pilot study A to determine the interstimulus interval for the discrimination task (ISI-d) and the interstimulus interval for the speech recognition task (ISI-r). Another two of these children participated in pilot study D, where the usability of training and testing modes were evaluated. Finally, one child completed the training in study IV, that is, 12 weeks of training regimes.

The inclusion criteria for the participants with CI were detailed below:

1. Prelingually deaf Malay Muslim children with CI.

2. Had at least 4 years of hearing experience with their implants.

3. Using auditory-verbal communication mode.

4. Attended mainstream school and religious classes (*Kelas Agama Fardu Ain: KAFA*) in the Malaysian Islamic Education curriculum to read the Holy Quran (at the time of the study).

5. They did not have any additional disabilities beside hearing impairment.

The exclusion criteria for the participants with CI were detailed below:

1. Those who were not using the Nucleus 24 cochlear implant system or its later generation.

2. Those with partial electrode insertion.

3.3.2 Control group (NH: Pilot studies B and C)

The study was advertised to recruit NH participants. They must fulfill the inclusion criteria below to participate in this study:

1. The child had normal hearing and speech development, as reported by the parents.

2. The child had no history of language disorders or learning difficulties.

3. Chronological age between 7 and 10 years old.

4. All Malay NH participants attended school & KAFA classes only and learned Arabic and Islamic education in the school following the national Islamic curriculum.

5. Native Arabic children relocated to Malaysia and learned in Arabic international school in Kuala Lumpur.

The demographic characteristics of study participants are summarized in **Table 3**.

3.4 Instrument, stimuli, and room calibration

Arabic Phonemes [/t/ ت], [/d/ د], [/k/ ك], and [/ʃ/ ش] were used in pilot study A, whereas [/ħ/ ح], [/sˤ/ ص], [/ðˤ/ ظ], and [/ʁ/ غ] were used in all other studies, that is, pilot studies B, C, and D and training study. All the phonemes were recorded and normalized for loudness-balanced. For more detail on stimuli preparation, see [6]. The conceptualized pathway shown in **Figure 1** was considered in designing the software. The design included both the discrimination and identification tasks. In both tasks, determining the optimum "distance" between the stimuli in a test track was important to ensure that participants with CI could hear the stimuli as two separate inputs.

3.5 Phase I: Determination of the interstimulus intervals (ISI)

In this experiment, the discrimination task was a two-alternative forced-choice (2AFC) task where stimuli were presented in pairs in the 'AX format. That is, two

S #	ID	C. Age	Nat	H. status	H. Age	Speech processor	Experiment	Study phase
1	C101	8 yrs.	M	CI	6 yrs.	Nucleus 5	pilot –A	Design
2	C102	10 yrs.	M	CI	8 yrs.	Nucleus 5	pilot –A	Design
3	A101	12 yrs.	A	NH	12 yrs.	NA	pilot –B	Design
4	A102	7 yrs.	A	NH	7 yrs.	NA	pilot –B	Design
5	N101	8 yrs.	M	NH	8 yrs.	NA	pilot –C	Development
6	N102	8 yrs.	M	NH	8 yrs.	NA	pilot –C	Development
7	N103	8 yrs.	M	NH	8 yrs.	NA	pilot –C	Development
8	N104	10 yrs.	M	NH	10 yrs.	NA	pilot –C	Development
9	N105	9 yrs.	M	NH	9 yrs.	NA	pilot –C	Development
10	CI-201	11 yrs.	M	CI	9 yrs.	Nucleus Freedom	pilot-D	Formative Evaluation
11	CI-203	7 yrs.	M	CI	4 yrs.	Nucleus 6	pilot-D	Formative Evaluation
12	CI-202	11 yrs.	M	CI	8 yrs.	Nucleus 6	pretest Training posttest	Implementation

Key: NA = not applicable; C. Age = Chronological Age; H. Age = hearing age; Nat = native; M = Malay; A = Arab.

Table 3.
Demographic characteristics of participants of the study and phase involved.

stimuli A (target sound) and stimuli X (minimal pair[1]) were presented with a very small ISI (300, 350, or 400 ms). The listener was required to judge whether the second stimulus presented was the *same or different* from the first stimulus. The *same* stimuli were presented in two forms, for example, /t/—/t/ and /d/—/d/, while *different* stimuli were presented as /t/—/d/ or /d/—/t/.

3.5.1 Preparation of the stimuli

The speech materials for pilot study A consisted of consonant-vowel (/Ca/) tokens with four Arabic phonemes/t, d, ʃ, and k/identified as familiar and better perceiving phonemes among the CI children [6]. The auditory stimuli for this experiment were further prepared by an open-source digital audio editor: Audacity version 2.1.3 for windows [77]. Two phonemes were put together in three different ISI-d (<, 500 ms), that is, 400 milliseconds (ms.), 350 ms., and 300 ms. for the discrimination task to activate bottom-up processing [48–51]. **Figure 3** illustrates ISI-d and ISI-r for both tasks.

An interstimulus interval for recognition (ISI-r), that is, 4000, 3500, 3000, or 2500 ms, was applied for each track. Therefore, three pairs of phonemes were presented in each presentation block with an ISI-d, for example, 400 ms., and an ISI-r, for example, 4000 ms. That generated 12 blocks of presentations: 12 blocks × 3 pairs of consonants x 3 ISI-d = 108 tokens for each combination pair. The details are shown in **Table 4**.

[1] In phonology a minimal pair of sound or phonemes differs in only one phonological feature, for example, /t/ & /d/ have same manner and place of articulation but differs only in voicing of articulation.

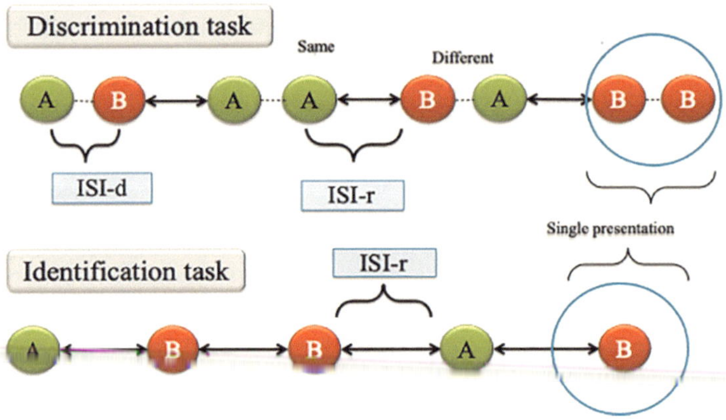

Figure 3.
Inter-stimulus-interval for discrimination (ISI-d) and intra-stimulus-interval for recognition (ISI-r) presentations.

Stimuli	Task (2AFC)	Presentation order	Numbers of presentation	ISI for presentations	Tokens per participant
/ʃ/–/k/	Discrimination	AB, BA	12 *Same* and 12 *Different* for each pair	ISI-d & ISI-r	1296
/t/–/d/		BB, AA			
/t/–/k/					
/ʃ/, /k/, /t/ & /d/	Identification	A & B	12 presentations for each stimulus	ISI-r	432

2AFC = Two alternative forced choice; ISI = Inter-stimulus interval; ISI-d = Inter-stimulus interval for discrimination; ISI-r = inter-stimulus interval for response in identification task.

Table 4.
Details of experimental paradigm for pilot study a to determine the best inter-stimulus intervals for discrimination (ISI-d) and identification (ISI-r) tasks.

3.5.2 Data collection

The participant was seated comfortably and was provided with the response sheet and a pencil. The stimuli were presented *via* a loudspeaker, positioned at approximately 30° azimuth and 1 m from the participant. The presentation level was around 65 dB SPL in an auditory alone mode. The tasks were verbally explained to the participant in the Malay language, and written instruction was given to parents. Before collecting data for the experiment *(discrimination and identification)*, participants were conditioned for each task. A total of 3456 tokens were collected from the two children with CI during the test presentation. The participants were tested using their CI with regularly used speech processor settings and programs.

3.5.3 Data analysis for pilot study A

The proportion of false alarms (pFA) was calculated using the equation (1). pFA is representative of response bias. The pFA was plotted on the graph against ISI-d and ISI-r for discrimination and identification tasks, respectively.

$$\text{pFA} = \frac{False\ alarms\ (FA)}{number\ of\ stimuli\ presented} \tag{1}$$

3.5.4 Results for pilot study A

Figure 4 illustrates the proportion of false alarm (pFA) at different interstimulus intervals tested during the discrimination and identification tasks. Overall, the ISI-d 350 ms for the discrimination task showed the lowest pFA (i.e., 0.09), and therefore selected for further study. For the identification task, different ISI-r did not affect the responses as response bias (pFA) was below (0.10–0.17). Therefore, 350 ms was chosen for ISI-d and 2500 ms for ISI-r.

3.6 Phase II: development of the *FizBil*© software

Following the determination of the ISI-d and ISI-r in pilot study A, these data were used in developing a software-based perceptual module named ***FizBil*©**. In this phase II of this study, ***FizBil*©** software was designed to engage non-native deaf listeners to attend to the perceptual cues and gradually learn categorical perception of non-native phonological features. It can be used as an experimental platform for the perceptual training of any sound stimuli.

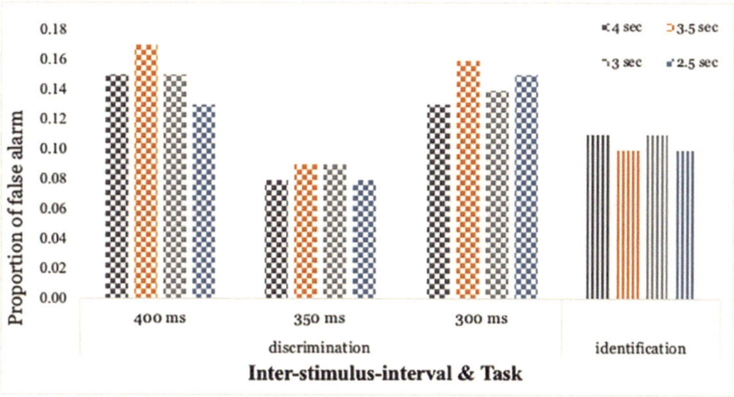

Figure 4.
Proportion of false alarm (pFA) at different test inter-stimulus intervals during the discrimination (ISI-d) and identification (ISI-r) tasks.

Figure 5.
Logo for FizBil® *in PNG (A) and vector file (B).*

An extensive literature review was done on perceptual training software and methodology. A one-to-one meeting was carried out between the software programmer and the researcher to discuss software design. ***FizBil***© was designed as a user-friendly platform. **Figure 5** shows the logo of the software.

3.6.1 Selection of phonemes for stimuli

The speech materials consist of the uncategorized-dispersed-assimilated Arabic phonemes [6] /ħ, sˤ, tˤ, ʁ/ in the consonant-vowel (a)- /Ca/ format. Each phoneme was paired with another phoneme that varies in a single phonological feature, that is, minimal pair (only one phonological component differs, wherever possible). For example, /t/ and /d/ are minimal pairs as they differ in voicing of articulation and have the same manner and place of articulation. **Table 5** presents the phoneme contrasts in each category.

3.6.2 Pilot study B

Pilot study B was conducted to check the program codes. Therefore, it is crucial to have listeners with minimal confusion and mature native perceptual space for all the phonological features. Test stimuli consist of emphatic sounds with secondary articulation and emphatic phonological features acquired later than nonemphatic cognates [47]. Therefore, native Arab children were invited to participate in this study. Two native Arabic-speaking NH children (aged 10 and 7 years) participated in pilot study B. Both participants (B-I and B-II) were siblings born in Egypt. Their father was working in one of the information technology-based companies, and they relocated to Kuala Lumpur two years back from the time of the study.

Phonemes	Phonological features	Minimal Pair for phonological-articulatory subcategories			Example of stimuli			
					Discrimination		Identification	
		Manner	Place	Voicing	Auditory	Visual display	Auditory	Visual Display
[/ħ/ح]	Pharyngeal, Fricative Voiceless	[/q/ق]	[/χ/ خ]	[/ʕ/ع]	χ – χ, ħ -ħ	Same	ħ - χ	خ & ح
					χ– ħ, ħ - χ	different		
[/ʁ/ غ]	Uvular Fricative Voiceless	[/q/ق]	[/ʕ/ ع]	[/χ/خ]	ʁ - ʁ, q-q	Same	ʁ - q	غ & ق
					ʁ - q, q - ʁ	different		
[/tˤ/ط]	Dental Plosive with Emphasis* Voiceless	[/sˤ/ص]	[/q/ ق]	[/dˤ/ض]	tˤ - tˤ, dˤ - dˤ	Same	tˤ & dˤ	ط &ض
					tˤ - dˤ, dˤ - tˤ	different		
[/sˤ/ص]	Alveolar Fricative with Emphasis* Voiceless	[/tˤ/ط]	[/ðˤ/ ظ]	[/dˤ/ض]	sˤ - sˤ, tˤ - tˤ	Same	sˤ & tˤ	ط & ص
					tˤ - sˤ, sˤ - tˤ	different		

**Secondary articulatory manner.*

Table 5.
Uncategorized-dispersed-assimilated Arabic consonants with their associated graphemes for Malay CI children and the corresponding minimal pairs used in the perceptual training.

The data were collected *via* the ***FizBil***© software. All responses from both participants were collected manually and concurrently auto-recorded on the notepad file by the software.

All the recorded responses (manually and notepad file) were compared to match the one-to-one score for the discrimination and identification tasks. The hit rate was calculated as the total correct responses.

3.6.2.1 Results

A total of 1440 (30 presentations × 3 minimal pairs for phonological features × 4 phonemes × 2 tasks × 2 participants) data tokens were collected from two Arabic-speaking participants with NH to check the program codes. The 1440 tokens were contained in a "notepad file" and coded by the researcher simultaneously. This method was adapted to check the responses in two ways.

The overall hit rate for the discrimination task was 99%, and the false alarm rate was 3% for both types of recording: notepad file and manual recording. However, for the identification task, the manual responses showed a hit rate of 98.0% with a 1% false alarm rate, while the miss rate and false alarm rate in the notepad file were 99%. These conflicts between the manual and notepad scoring suggest a coding mistake in the software writing. Therefore, the software was reverted to the software programmer and debugged accordingly. The identification test was repeated as this part of the software was debugged. Thus, another 720 tokens were recollected and reanalyzed. As a result, the overall hit rate for the identification task was 98.3%, and the false alarm rate was 2% for both notepad and manual note files. Thus, the ***FizBil***© revised coding for the identification task was accepted.

3.7 Phase III: formative evaluation of the FizBil© software

3.7.1 Pilot study C

Pilot study C was designed to explore the interface usability for children after minimizing controlling variables such as perceptual difficulties. Unfamiliar phonemes [/ħ/, ح] were used as stimuli in this pilot study.

Five Malay NH children (age: Range = 8–10 years; Mean = 8.6 years; Standard deviation = 0.9 years) who fulfilled the inclusion criteria participated.

The tests were conducted in a quiet room at their own homes using the *FizBil*© software. Stimuli were presented from a loudspeaker connected to the laptop at a comfortably loud level.

All collected responses from pilot study C were compared, that is, discrimination task manual scores vs. notepad scores. In addition, a correct percentage score of the hit rate was calculated.

3.7.1.1 Results

A total of 900 (30 presentations × 3 minimal pairs for phonological feature × 1 phoneme × 2 tasks × 5 participants) tokens were collected during pilot C from five NH Malay children during the discrimination and identification tasks consonant /ħ/. The hit rate was 99.7% for the discrimination task, while the hit rate for the identification task was 97%. These relatively high performances for both tests suggested that they were relatively easy for NH children. However, due to the ceiling performances of the participants, the d-prime score (d') was not calculated.

3.7.2 Phase III: pilot study D

Pilot study D was conducted on native Malay children with CI to examine the overall suitability of user interface and instruction.

Two CI children participated, aged 11 and 8 years, with hearing ages nine and 4 years, respectively. They used a Cochlear Nucleus N6 speech processor with the *Advanced Combination Encoder (ACE)* speech processing strategy and audio-verbal communication mode. Both participants attended mainstream schools.

The stimuli (phonemes /ħ, sˤ, tˤ, ʁ/: detail in **Table 4**) were used in this pilot study and were presented *via* the *FizBil*© software installed in window laptop. The data were collected at the Audiology clinic of UKM. Data for both listening conditions, that is, with and without feedback, were collected for 80–90 minutes a week intervals.

Overall, 2880 tokens (30 presentations × 3 minimal pairs for phonological feature x 4 phonemes × 2 tasks × 2 participants × 2 modes, i.e., with and without feedback) were collected and analyzed. The hit rate was 78%, and the false alarm rate was 22%. Therefore, the d' scores were calculated.

The d' score is the perceptual peak difference between two signals. Mathematically, it is the difference between the standard deviation (z-score) corresponding to the proportion of hit rate and false alarm rate. Equation (ii) was used to calculate the d' scores as an index of perception.

$$d' = z(pH) - z(pFA) \quad (2)$$

3.7.2.1 Results

The bar graph (**Figure 6**) illustrates the d' scores of two CI participants for four unfamiliar Arabic phonemes in two testing conditions. In the first condition,

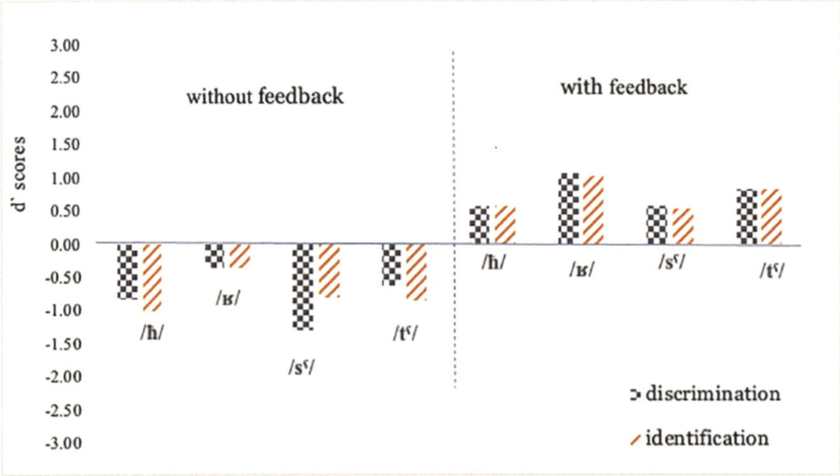

Figure 6.
Comparison of the perceptual learning scores (d') of uncategorized-dispersed-assimilated Arabic consonants with and without feedback in both the discrimination and identification tasks.

that is, without feedback, perceptual confusions for all four unfamiliar phonemes were evident. The relatively low d' scores for /ħ, sˤ, tˤ, ʁ/ were – 1.0, −0.5, −1.5, and 0.75, respectively. In the second testing condition, all listening stimuli were paired with feedback. A dramatic rise was detected in perceptual scores of four unfamiliar Arabic phonemes. The positive d' scores for /ħ, sˤ, tˤ, ʁ/ were evidence. Hence, the feedback interface was user-friendly and could be used for perceptual training.

3.8 Phase IV: perceptual training—a case study

Phase IV is a pre-post training experimental design conducted over 12 weeks. Only three out of seven CI children invited and consented by their parents to participate. However, out of these three children, one child only participated in the pretest, while the second child dropped off after the second training session. Hence, the data were from only one participant who completed all sessions.

The training design is shown in **Figure 7**. Baseline responses were collected during pre-training on week 1. Then, from weeks 2 to 5, categorical perceptual training with feedback was provided for manner, place, and voicing categories. The training was done once a week. In each training session, 30 stimuli of each phoneme for each phonological category were presented in discrimination and identification tasks [(30 presentations × 3 phonological features × 2 tasks) × 4 phonemes/session]. Therefore, each phoneme was heard 180 times in three different minimal pairs per training session. Moreover, 720 stimuli were presented per visit. In total, 2880 stimuli were presented to the participant in 4 weeks of training. Each training session

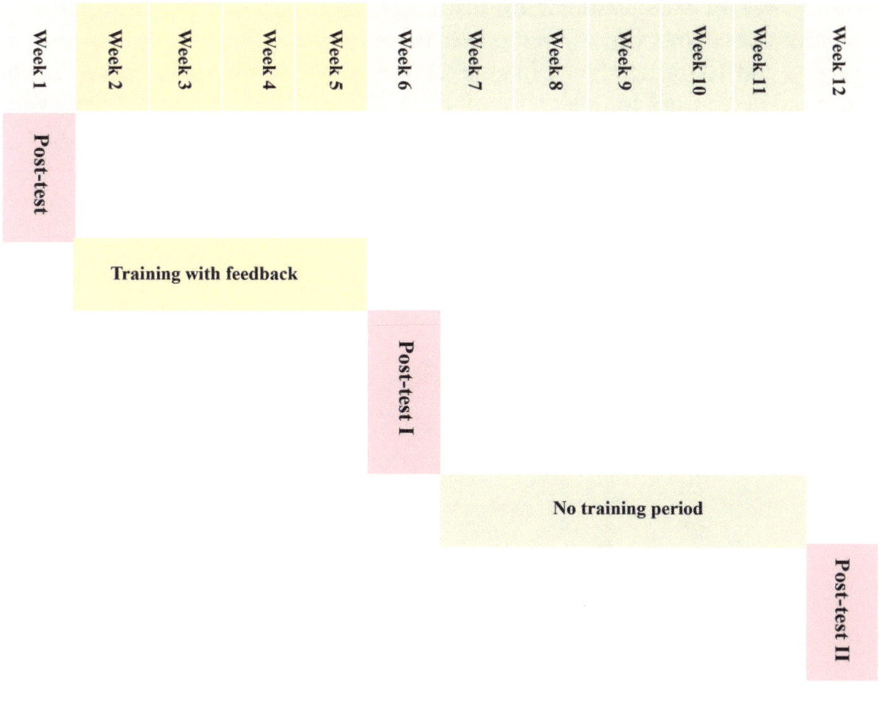

Figure 7.
The 12-week perceptual training and test regime used in this study.

lasted approximately 70–90 minutes (mins.), including two 5-minute forced breaks after 20–25 mins. The post-tests I and II (maintenance) data were collected at weeks six and 12.

During pretest (baseline) and post-tests I and II, a total of 2160 tokens were collected. This data was analyzed according to the SDT recommendations for pretest and post-test. The d-prime (d') scores were calculated to measure perceptual learning of phonological features' discrimination and identification before and after the training. The negative d' score indicates perceptual confusion. A positive value of d' score represents the perceptual category in the perceptual space [52–55].

3.8.1 Overall perceptual learning effect

Figure 8 shows the perceptual learning effect of dispersed uncategorized assimilated phonemes. Bars at the left present the child's baseline (week 1) perceptual ability. The participant had perceptual confusion, as indicated by the negative d' values for all the tested uncategorized assimilated Arabic phonemes. However, the d' scores improved after 4 weeks of training and were retained after five weeks of no-training period. Positive d' values seen at post-test I indicate a sharpening of the perceptual categories for all the uncategorized-dispersed-assimilated Arabic phonemes. The positive d' scores remained at post-test II, suggesting the learning effect and concrete conceptualization were evidence.

3.8.2 Perceptual learning for phonological categories

The effect of training and perceptual learning was further explored by comparing the mean scores for each phonological feature at baseline, post-test I, and post-test II for posterior consonants (/ħ, ʁ/) and emphatic consonants (/sˤ, tˤ/). Results are shown in **Figures 9** and **10**, respectively. In general, it has been found that at baseline, the child showed perceptual confusion for all three phonological categories. However, post-training, perceptual learning occurred as indicated by the positive d' values. At

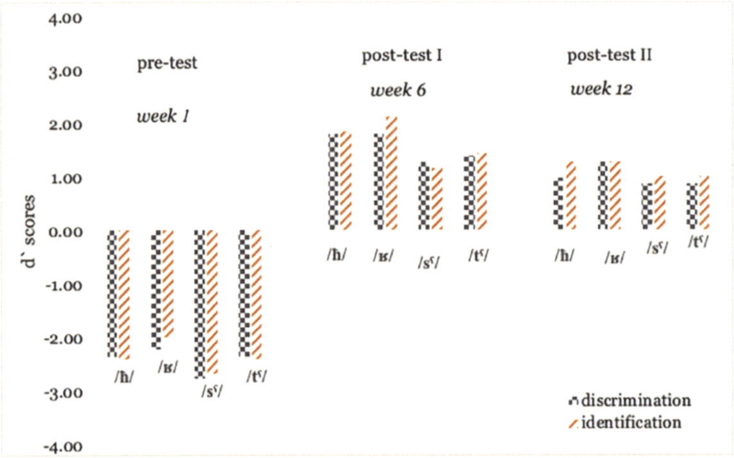

Figure 8.
The overall perceptual learning effects for uncategorized-dispersed-assimilated Arabic phonemes in discrimination and identification tasks in a Malay child with CI.

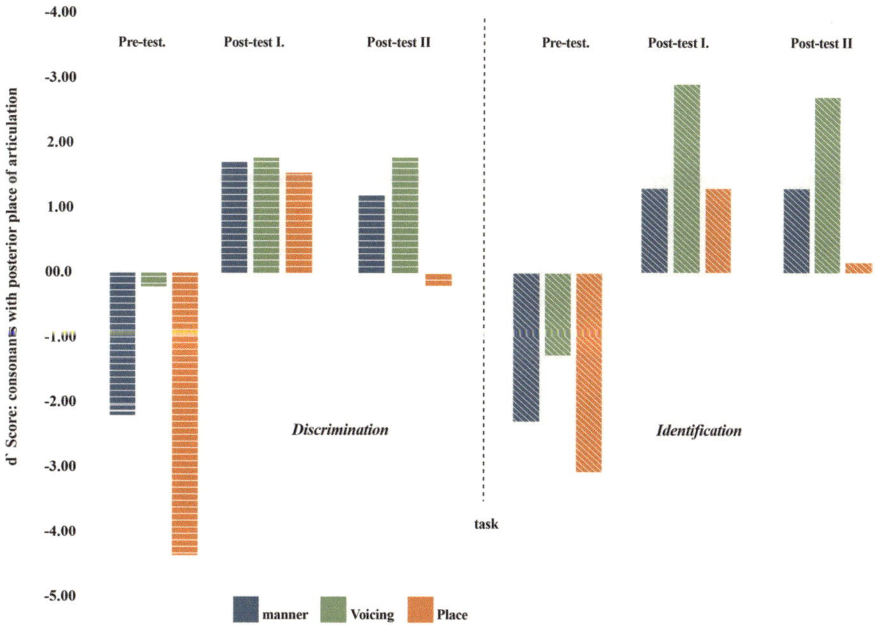

Figure 9.
The perceptual learning effects based on phonological features for uncategorized-dispersed-assimilated Arabic posterior place of articulation.

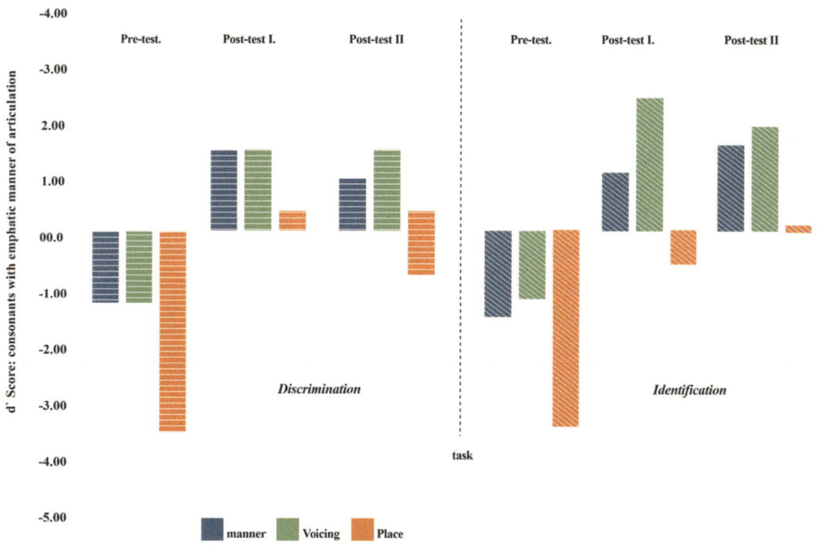

Figure 10.
The perceptual learning effects based on phonological features for uncategorized-dispersed-assimilated Arabic emphatic manner of articulation.

post-test II, while retention was observed for manner and voicing, the place of articulation suffered after five weeks of the no-training period. The results were similar for both discrimination and identification tasks for both posterior (see **Figure 9**) and emphatic consonants (see **Figure 10**).

4. Discussion

This study examined the perceptual learning of uncategorized-dispersed-assimilated Arabic consonants for a group of non-native children with CI using a newly developed, *FizBil*© bottom-up, customized software training module. The design and development of the *FizBil*© software, which was based on the signal detection theory, have been described in detail, involving identification and discrimination task modules. **Figure 2** shows the hypothetical pathway of signal detection and non-native phonemes' assimilation, involving top-down and bottom-up signal processing. This figure serves as the framework for this study.

4.1 Perceptual learning

Non-native perceptual difficulties are solely based on native language effects arising from the sharpening of perceptual categories [37] during language acquisition. New category learning and the sharpening of learned perceptual categories depend on bottom-up processing. Bottom-up perceptual training occurs when auditory stimuli are presented with small intervals, that is, less than a second [66, 67, 78–83]. However, most non-native and auditory training regimes are based on identification tasks. On the other hand, a CI device provides more access to the envelope and temporal cues than the spectral information of sound signal [28, 29, 49, 84]. Therefore, discrimination training should be added alongside identification training.

It should be noted that previous studies have indicated that production is directly correlated with the perception of both native [62, 85] and non-native [36–46, 70–76] phonological features. However, studies on improving the perceptual peaks or perceiving distinct phonological boundaries among non-native children with CI have yet to be reported. Thus, the design, development, and evaluation of the *FizBil*© software described in this chapter are meant explicitly for this training purpose.

According to the signal detection theory (SDT), the perception of a phoneme is a twofold process that comprises sensory processing and decision-making [52–56]. SDT provides the psychophysical measure of information processing that enables listeners to distinguish between information-bearing patterns and recognize them as two separate entities [47, 86, 87]. Research studies have shown that non-native perceptual difficulties of NH adults [36–39, 41, 43–46, 69–71, 74–76, 79, 80] and children [88] are solely based on native language phonological repertoire. These effects arise from sharpening perceptual categories [37] during language acquisition [51, 89]. Nonetheless, for CI children, we need to consider information transmission *via* the cochlear implant device on top of the communication for signal processing and assimilated perception of non-native phonemes [6, 8–22, 35].

Kolb's experiential learning theory (KELT) model defines that learning occurs with experience, and learners have different abilities to acquire knowledge or information [90, 91]. Experiential learning can only happen when teaching and instructional design is carefully chosen [92]. Kolb [93] has explained that the four-stage experiential learning cycle starts with the concrete experience, followed by reflective observation, abstract conceptualization, and actively trying out. According to KELT, learners have learning style preferences. Self-evaluation is a primary component in KELT that provides learners with feedback training. **Figure 11** represents the conceptualized framework for perceptual learning of non-native phonemes and training task effects.

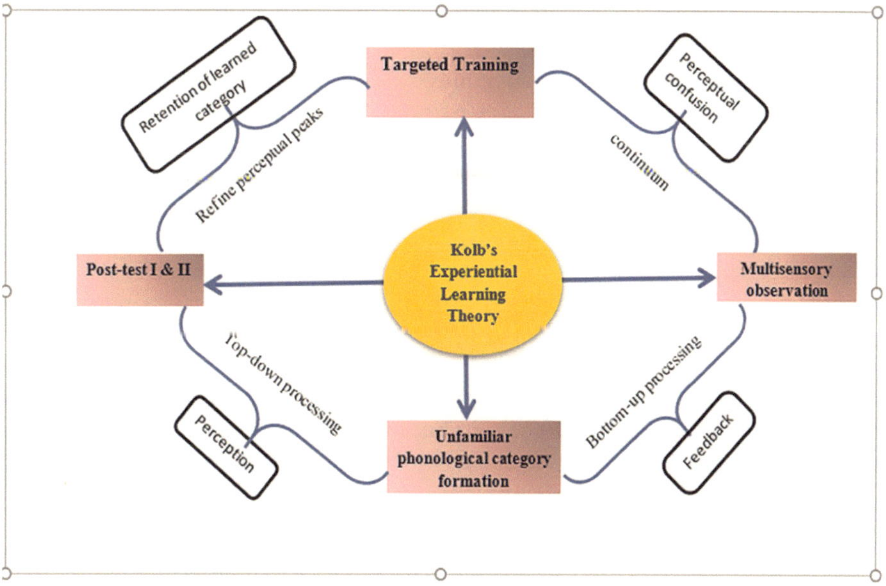

Figure 11.
The conceptualized framework for perceptual learning of non-native phonemes and training task effects based on the KELT model.

The perceptual training study evaluated the ***FizBil***© software developed with specific ISI-d and ISI-r for testing children with CI based on the bottom-up information processing model. Only one child out of three volunteers who participated completed the 12-week training and test regime. Thus, the data reported was from a Malay CI child with 2160 tokens collected. While this limits the researcher from generalizing the finding, the results from one participant are still worth to discuss as the tokens collected were huge. However, given that the main aim of phase IV was to implement the ***FizBil***© software, it was evident that the newly developed training software was valuable and could be used for training purposes. As evidenced by the findings, the perception of confusing Arabic phonemes could be sharpened into the three phonological categories following training. Results are discussed below based on the KELT theoretical framework.

KELT defines the theoretical and practical elements for a learner-centered approach [90–92]. It is a cycle of four components: reflecting, thinking, acting, and experiencing [90, 92, 94]. Learning is a multilayered process that includes multisensory information processing. Processing occurs in two ways, that is, reflective observation and active experimentation. On the other hand, perception occurs with concrete experience and abstract conceptualization. The feedback during the training in the present study provided active experimentation (discrimination and identification in minimal pairs) and built the abstract conceptualization in the perceptual space with substantial experience [95–97].

At baseline, within the Malay perceptual space of the CI child, there was the no-category formation of phonological features for posterior unfamiliar (**Figure 9** baseline) and emphatic (**Figure 10** baseline) Arabic phonemes. The d' scores showed negative values. However, four weeks of bottom-up training resulted in absolute manner, place, and voicing of articulation category formation for posterior and emphatic unfamiliar Arabic phonemes (see **Figures 9** and **10**). It could be observed that the learning effects for manner and voicing of articulation features were more prominent than the place of articulation.

In speech signals, the envelope cues convey the voicing and manner features, that is, the slow periodic waves [88]. CI processing deficit in spectral cues transmission could explain why CI users struggle with place feature learning [30, 33, 34]. Spectral cues processing insufficiency is partly due to the limitation in their electrode discrimination abilities [28–31, 84, 98]. All the factors mentioned above affect the perception of the place of articulation among CI children. That might be part of the reason for the place feature category decline after five weeks of the no-training period, which probably requires a little more time to sharpen the perceptual peak. In other words, the overall d' scores decline in post-test II (**Figures 9** and **10**) could be due to place feature learning effect decay. However, the findings showed that the learning effects of manner and voice articulation were sustained after the long five weeks of off-training, as indicated by the blue and green bars in **Figures 9** and **10**. In post-test II, the identification of phonological features was better than discrimination. Discrimination task is exclusively based on short-term memory and carried out auditorily [33, 81–83, 98, 99]. In a short time (100–500 ms), one has to discriminate the two sounds [49, 53, 56, 61, 92, 99–101]. This discrepancy might be due to information transmission difficulties using the cochlear implant hearing device [30, 35, 98].

5. Conclusion

In this study, the perceptual learning effects were evidenced using the bottom-up training and led to category formation in the perceptual space of the non-native child with CI. Phonological categories breakdown analyses revealed that manner and voicing feature category formation emerged after four weeks of training and was retained after five weeks of off-training. In contrast, place feature formation, observed after four weeks of training in both discrimination and identification tasks, declined after five weeks of the off-training period, suggesting more extended and ongoing training might be needed for the perception of place features. Further analyses revealed that the perceptual learning effects of the posterior place of articulation were less than the emphatic manner of articulation. The learning effects of emphatic manner were retained after five weeks of off-training, whereas the posterior place perceptual learning effect noticeably declined. In conclusion, the perception of uncategorized-dispersed-assimilated Arabic consonants could be refined within the Malay perceptual space by bottom-up training in congenitally deaf, non-native CI children.

Author details

Farheen Naz Anis and Cila Umat*
Faculty of Health Sciences, Center for Rehabilitation and Special Needs Studies, Universiti Kebangsaan Malaysia, Kuala Lumpur, Malaysia

*Address all correspondence to: cila@ukm.edu.my

References

[1] Geers AE, Niparko JK, Geers AE. Speech, language, and reading skills after early cochlear implantation. Journal of the American Medical Association. 2004; **291**(19):2378-2380

[2] Geers AE, Nicholas JG, Sedey AL. Language skills of children with early Cochlear implantation. Ear and Hearing. 2003;**24**:46-58

[3] Geers AE, Nicholas J, Tobey E, Davidsonb L. Language emergence in early-implanted children. Journal of Speech, Language, and Hearing Research. 2016;**59**(2):155-170

[4] Geers A, Brenner C, Nicholas J, Uchanski R, Tye-Murray N, Tobey E. Rehabilitation factors contributing to implant benefit in children. The Annals of Otology, Rhinology, and Laryngology. 2002;**111**:127-130

[5] Goh B, Fadzilah N, Abdullah A, Fathi B, Umat C. Long-term outcomes of Universiti Kebangsaan Malaysia Cochlear implant program among pediatric implantees. International Journal of Pediatric Otorhino-laryngology. 2018;**105**(September 2017): 27-32

[6] Anis FN, Umat C, Ahmad K, Hamid BA. Patterns of recognition of Arabic consonants by non-native children with cochlear implants and normal hearing. Cochlear Implants International. 2019; **20**(1):1-11

[7] Anis FN, Umat C, Ahmad K, Hamid BA. Arabic place feature confusions among severely and profoundly hearing impaired children with a cochlear implant. In: 4th International Conference on Social Sciences Research 2016 (ICSSR 2016). 2016. pp. 207-216

[8] Bunta FC, Elizabeth G-M, Procter A, Hernandeza A. Initial stop voicing in bilingual children with Cochlear implants and their typically developing peers with Normal hearing. J speech, Lang. Hearing Research. 2016;**59** (August):686-698

[9] Delcenserie A, Genesee F, Trudeau N, Champoux F. The development of phonological memory and language: A multiple groups approach. Journal of Child Language. 2020;**48**(2): 285-324

[10] Nassif N, Barezzani MG, Oscar L, De ZR. Delayed speech perception and production after Cochlear implantation in bilingual children from non-native families. Journal of Otorhinolaryngology, Hearing and Balance Medicine. 2021;**2**(1):4

[11] Sosa AV, Bunta F. Speech production accuracy and variability in monolingual and bilingual children with cochlear implants: A comparison to their peers with normal hearing. Journal of Speech, Language, and Hearing Research. 2019; **62**(8):2601-2616

[12] Keilmann A, Friese B, Hoffmann V. Receptive and productive speech and language abilities in hearing-impaired children with German as a second language. International Journal of Pediatric Otorhinolaryngology. 2019; **120**:100-107

[13] Rødvik AK, Tvete O, von Torkildsen JK, OBØ W, Skaug I, Silvola JT. Consonant and vowel confusions in well-performing children and adolescents with cochlear implants, measured by a nonsense syllable repetition test. Frontiers in Psychology. 2019;**10**(AUG): 1-17

[14] Thomas E, El-Kashlan H, Zwolan TA. Children with cochlear implants who live in monolingual and bilingual homes. Otology & Neurotology. 2008 Feb;**29**(2):230-234

[15] Waltzman SB, Robbins AMC, Green JE, Cohen NL. Second oral language capabilities in children with cochlear implants. Otology and Neurotology. 2003;**24**(5):757-763

[16] Mahon M, Vickers D, McCarthy K, Barker R, Merritt R, Szagun G, et al. Cochlear-implanted children from homes where english is an additional language: Findings from a recent audit in one London Centre. Cochlear Implants International. 2011;**12**(2):105-113

[17] McKee RL. The construction of deaf children as marginal bilinguals in the mainstream. International Journal of Bilingual Education and Bilingualism. 2008;**11**(5):519-540

[18] Bunta F, Douglas M. The effects of dual-language support on the language skills of bilingual children with hearing loss who use listening devices relative to their monolingual peers. Language, Speech, and Hearing Services in Schools. 2013;**44**(3):281-290

[19] Bunta F, Douglas M, Dickson H, Cantu A, Wickesberg J, Gifford RH. Dual language versus English only support for bilingual children with hearing loss who use cochlear implants and hearing aids. International Journal of Language & Communication Disorders. 2016;**51**(4):460-472

[20] Sabri M, Fabiano-Smith L. Phonological development in a bilingual Arabic–english-speaking child with bilateral cochlear implants: A longitudinal case study. American Journal of Speech-Language Pathology. 2018;**27**(4):1506-1522

[21] Forli F, Giuntini G, Ciabotti A, Bruschini L, Löfkvist U, Berrettini S. How does a bilingual environment affect the results in children with cochlear implants compared to monolingual-matched children? An Italian follow-up study. International Journal of Pediatric Otorhinolaryngology. 2018;**2018**(105):56-62

[22] Deriaz M, Pelizzone M, Fornos AP. Simultaneous development of 2 oral languages by child cochlear implant recipients. Otology & Neurotology. 2014;**35**(9):1541-1544

[23] Abdul-Kadir NA, Sudirman R. Difficulties of standard Arabic phonemes spoken by non-Arab primary school children based on formant frequencies. Journal of Computer Science. 2011;**7**(7):1003-1010

[24] Azraai H. Acoustic analysis of Al-Quran phonemes by children with cochlear implant. In: poster. Malaysia: UNIVERSITI KEBANGSAAN MALAYSIA; 2011

[25] Teschendorf M, Arweiler-Harbeck D, Bagus H. Speech development after cochlear implantation in children with bilingual parents. Cochlear Implants International. 2010;**11**(Suppl 1):386-389

[26] Teschendorf M, Janeschik S, Bagus H, Lang S, Arweiler-Harbeck D. Speech development after cochlear implantation in children from bilingual homes. Cochlear Implants International. 2011;**32**(2):229-235

[27] Clark G. In: Beyer RT, editor. Cochlear Implants: Fundamentals and Application [Internet]. New York, NY: Springer; 2003. 243 p

[28] Shannon RV, Fu Q-J, Galvin J. The number of spectral channels required for speech recognition depends

on the difficulty of the listening situation. Acta oto-laryngologica Suppl. 2004;**552**:50-54

[29] Shannon RV, Fu Q-J, Galvin J, Friesen L. Speech perception with Cochlear implants. In: Cochlear Implants: Auditory Prostheses and Electric Hearing SE - 8. 2004. pp. 334-376

[30] Verschuur C. Acoustic Model of Consonant Recognition in Cochlear Implant Users [thesis]. England: University of Southampton; 2007

[31] Zhou N, Xu L, Lee C-Y. The effects of frequency-place shift on consonant confusion in cochlear implant simulations. Journal of the Acoustical Society of America. 2010;**128**(1):401-409

[32] Bouton S, Colé P, Serniclaes W. The influence of lexical knowledge on phoneme discrimination in deaf children with cochlear implants. Speech Communication. 2012;**54**(2):189-198

[33] Moreno-Torres I, Moruno-López E, Ignacio M-T, Moruno-López E. Segmental and suprasegmental errors in Spanish learning cochlear implant users: Neurolinguistic interpretation. Journal of Neurolinguistics. 2014;**31**:1-16

[34] Bouton S, Serniclaes W, Bertoncini J, Cole P. Perception of speech features by French-speaking children with Cochlear implants. Journal of Speech, Language, and Hearing Research. 2012;**55**(1):139-153

[35] Nittrouer S, Caldwell-Tarr A, Moberly AC, Lowenstein JH. Perceptual weighting strategies of children with cochlear implants and normal hearing. Pediatric Cochlear Implantation. 2014; **52**:111-133

[36] Best CT, Strange W. Effects of phonological and phonetic factors on cross language perception of approximants. Journal of Phonetics. 1992;**110**:89-108

[37] Best CT, Goldstein LM, Nam H, Tyler MD, Best CT, Goldstein LM, et al. Articulating what infants attune to in native speech. Ecological Psychology. 2016;**28**(4):216-261

[38] Evans BG, Alshangiti W. The perception and production of British English vowels and consonants by Arabic learners of English. Journal of Phonetics. 2018;**68**:15-31

[39] Faris MM, Best CT, Tyler MD. An examination of the different ways that non-native phones may be perceptually assimilated as uncategorized. Journal of the Acoustical Society of America. 2016; **139**(January):1-5

[40] Faris MM, Best CT, Tyler MD. Discrimination of uncategorised non-native vowel contrasts is modulated by perceived overlap with native phonological categories. Journal of Phonetics. 2018;**70**(July):1-19

[41] Dommelen WA, Hazan V. Perception of English consonants in noise by native and Norwegian listeners. Speech Communication. 2010;**52**(11–12): 968-979

[42] Brown CA. The role of the L1 grammar in the L2 acquisition of segmental structure. Second Language Research. 1998;**14**(2):136-193

[43] Best CT, Tyler MD. Nonnative and second language speech perception. Commonalities and complementarities, in second language speech learning: The role of language experience in speech perception and production. In: Munro MJ, Bohn OS, editors. Language

Experience in Second Language Speech Learning. Amsterdam: John Benjamins; 2007. pp. 13-34

[44] Best CT, Goldstein L, Tyler MD, Nam H. Articulating the perceptual assimilation model (PAM): Perceptual assimilation in relation to articulatory organs and their constriction gestures. The Journal of the Acoustical Society of America. 2009; **125**:2758

[45] Best CT, Hallé P, a. Perception of initial obstruent voicing is influenced by gestural organization. Journal of Phonetics. 2010;**38**(1):109-126

[46] Georgiou GP, Perfilieva NV, Denisenko VN, Novospasskaya NV. Perceptual realization of Greek consonants by Russian monolingual speakers. Speech Communication. 2020; **125**(September):7-14

[47] Silbert NH. Perception of voicing and place of articulation in labial and alveolar English stop consonants. Laboratory Phonology. 2014;**5**(2):289-335

[48] Lo CY, McMahon CM, Looi V, Thompson WF. Melodic contour training and its effect on speech in noise, consonant discrimination, and prosody perception for Cochlear implant recipients. Behavioural Neurology. 2015. pp. 10. [Article No: 352869]

[49] Gerrits E, Schouten MEH. Categorical perception depends on the discrimination task. Perception & Psychophysics. 2004;**66**(3):363-376

[50] Wang X, Humes LE. Classification and cue weighting of multidimensional stimuli with speech-like cues for young normal hearing and elderly hearing-impaired listeners. Ear Hear. 2008;**29**(5): 725-745

[51] Pajak B, Levy R. The role of abstraction in non-native speech perception. Journal of Phonetics. 2014; **46**(1):147-160

[52] Harvey LO, Parker SM. Detection theory: Sensory and decision processes. In: Psychology of Perception. Boulder: Colorado University. 2014

[53] Macmillan NA, Creelmen CD. Detection Theory: A user's Guide. Second ed. New York, NY: Psychology Press; 2005

[54] Georgeson M. Postgraduate research methods course. In: Sensitivity and Bias - an Introduction to Signal Detection Theory. UK: University of Birmingham; 2005

[55] Stanislaw H, Todorov N. Calculation of signal detection theory measures. Behavior Research Methods, Instruments, & Computers. 1999;**31**(1): 137-149

[56] Ashby F, Soto F. Multidimensional signal detection theory. In: Townsend Z, Wang AE, editors. Oxford Handbook of Computational and Mathematical Psychology. UK: Oxford University Press; 2012

[57] Handley Z, Moore D. Training novel phonemic contrasts: A comparison of identification and oddity discrimination training. Proc SLaTE. 2009;**2**:3-6

[58] Huyse A, Berthommier F, Leybaert J. Degradation of labial information modifies audiovisual speech perception in cochlear-implanted children. Ear and Hearing. 2012;**34**(1):110-121

[59] Jaekel BN, Newman RS, Goupell MJ. Speech rate normalization and phonemic

boundary perception in cochlear-implant users. Journal of Speech, Language, and Hearing Research. 2017; **60**(5):1398-1416

[60] Lesniak A, Myers L, Dodd B. The English phonological awareness skills of 5;0-6;0-year-old polish–English, Portuguese–English bilingual speakers and English monolingual children. Speech, Language and Hearing. 2014;**17** (1):37-48

[61] Moore DR, Rosenberg JF, Coleman JS. Discrimination training of phonemic contrasts enhances phonological processing in mainstream school children. Brain and Language. 2005;**94** (1):72-85

[62] Holt LL, Lotto AJ. Speech perception as categorization. Attention, Perception, Psychophys. 2010;**72**(5): 1218-1227

[63] Heeren WFL. Perceptual development of phoneme contrasts in adults and children [Internet]. 2006. Available from: http://igitur-archive.library.uu.nl/dissertations/2006-0712-200026/UUindex.html.

[64] Serniclaes W, Sprenger-Charolles L. Categorical perception of speech sounds and dyslexia. Current Psychology Letters. 2003;**10**(1):1-9

[65] Reed MA. Speech perception and the discrimination of brief auditory cues in Reading disabled children. Journal of Experimental Child Psychology. 1989; **48**:270-292

[66] Pisoni DB, Kronenberger WG, Chandramouli SH, Conway CM. Learning and memory processes following cochlear implantation: The missing piece of the puzzle. Frontiers in Psychology. 2016; **7**(APR):1-19

[67] Pisoni DD, Geers AE. Working memory in deaf children with cochlear implants: Correlations between digit span and measures of spoken language processing. The Annals of Otology, Rhinology & Laryngology. Supplement. 2000;**185**(December):89-92

[68] APA. What is Learned in Perceptual Learning? [Internet]. American Psychological Association. 2013. Available from: https://www.apa.org/pubs/highlights/peeps/issue-04.

[69] Best CT, McRoberts GW, Goodell E. Discrimination of non-native consonant contrasts varying in perceptual assimilation to the listener's native phonological system. The Journal of the Acoustical Society of America. 2001;**109** (2):775-794

[70] Flege JE. Phonetic approximation in second language acquisition. Language Learning. 1980;**30**(1):117-134

[71] Flege JE, Munro MJ, Mackay IR, a. Effects of age of second-language learning on the production of English consonants. Speech Communication. 1995;**16**(1):1-26

[72] Polka L. Cross-language speech perception in adults: Phonemic, phonetic, and acoustic contributions. Journal of the Acoustical Society of America. 1991;**89**(6):2961-2977

[73] Werker JFF, Lalonde CEE. Cross-language speech perception: Initial capabilities and developmental change. Developmental Psychology. 1988;**24**(5): 672-683

[74] Ritchie WC. On the explanation of phonic interference. Language Learn. 1968;**18**(3–4):183-197

[75] Werker JF, Tees RC. Cross-language speech perception: Evidence for

perceptual reorganization during the first year of life. Infant Behavior & Development. 2002;**25**(1):121-133

[76] Hancin-Bhatt BJ. Phonological Transfer in Seecond Language Perception and Production [thesis]. USA: University of Illinois; 1994

[77] Mazzoni D, Dannenberg R. Audacity Credit. Addacity team; 2000

[78] Bradlow AR, Akahane-yamada R. Training Japanese listeners to identify English /r/ and /l/: Long term retention of learning in perception and production. Perception & Psychophysics. 1999;**61**(5):977-985

[79] Bradlow AR, Pisoni DB. Some effects of perceptual learning on speech production. The Journal of the Acoustical Society of America. 1997;**101**(4):2299-2310

[80] Pisoni DB, Remez RE. The Handbook of Speech Perception. Oxford, UK: Blackwell Publishing; 2006

[81] Pisoni DB. Auditory short-term memory and vowel perception. Memory and Cognition. 1975;**6**(8):1-25

[82] Pisoni DB. Auditory and phonetic memory codes in the discrimination of consonants and vowels. Perception & Psychophysics. 1973;**13**(1):1-23

[83] Pisoni DB, Kronenberger WG, Harris MS, Moberly AC. Three challenges for future research on cochlear implants. The World Journal of Otorhinolaryngology – Head & Neck Surgery. 2017;**12**(10):1-15

[84] Li F. Perceptual Cues of Consonant Sound and Impact of Sensorineural Hearing Loss on Speech Perception. USA: University of Illinois; 2009

[85] Casserly ED, Pisoni DB. Speech perception and production. Wiley Interdisciplinary Reviews: Cognitive Science. 2010;**1**(5):629

[86] Abdi H. Signal detection theory. In: International Encyclopedia of Education. Vol. March. 2010

[87] Stoehr A, Benders T, van Hell JG, Fikkert P. Bilingual Preschoolers' speech is associated with non-native maternal language input. Language Learning and Development. 2019;**15**(1):75-100

[88] Driscoll VD, Oleson J, Dingfeng Jiang A, Gfeller K. Effects of training on recognition of musical instruments presented through Cochlear implant simulations. Journal of the American Academy of Audiology. 2009;**20**(1):71-82

[89] Melguy YV. Exploring the bilingual phonological space: Early Bilinguals' discrimination of coronal stop contrasts. Language and Speech. 2017;**61**(2):173-198

[90] Kang DY, Martin SN. Improving learning opportunities for special education needs (SEN) students by engaging pre-service science teachers in an informal experiential learning course. Asia Pacific Journal of Education. 2018;**38**(3):319-347

[91] Kolb DA, Boyatzis RE, Mainemelis C. Experiential learning theory: Previous research and new directions. Perspect Thinking, Learning and Cognitive Styles. 2000;**216**:227-247

[92] Wright BA, Zhang Y. A review of the generalization of auditory learning. Philosophical Transactions of the Royal Society B. 2009;**364**(1515):301-311

[93] Kolb D. In: NPH EC, editor. Experiential Learning: Experience as the

Source of Learning and Development. Prentice-Hall; 1984

[94] Wright J. Experiential Learning: An Overview. Institute for Teaching and Learning Innovations. Brisbane: University of Queensland; 2015. p. 8

[95] Miller V. Learn, Try, Repeat: Experiential Learning in Adult Second Language Acquisition of Spanish in Higher Education [thesis]. USA: University of Nebraska – Lincoln; 2021

[96] Reimer CK. The Effect of Retrieval Practice on Vocabulary Learning for Children Who Are Deaf or Hard of Hearing. USA: Washington University; 2019

[97] Baker MA. The Effect of Kolb's Experiential Learning Model on Successful Secondary Student Intelligence and Student Motivation [thesis]. Oklahoma: Oklahoma State University; 2012

[98] Shannon RV, Cruz RJ, Galvin JJ, Galvin JJ 3rd. Effect of stimulation rate on Cochlear implant Users' phoneme , word and sentence recognition in quiet and in noise. Audiology and Neurotology. 2011;**16**:113-123

[99] Watson DR, Titterington J, Henry A, Toner JG. Auditory sensory memory and working memory processes in children with normal hearing and cochlear implants. Audiology and Neurotology. 2007;**12**(2):65-76

[100] Zhang YX, Moore DR, Guiraud J, Molloy K, Yan TT, Amitay S. Auditory discrimination learning: Role of working memory. PLoS One. 2016;**11**(1):1-18

[101] Kasisopa B, Antonios LEK, Jongman A, Sereno JA, Burnham D. Training children to perceive non-native lexical tones: Tone language background, bilingualism, and auditory-visual information. Frontiers in Psychology. 2018;**9**(9):1508

Chapter 7

Perspective Chapter: Cochlear Implant Activation in the Immediate Postoperative Period at the Operating Room

Gislaine Richter Minhoto Wiemes,
Nicole Richter Minhoto Wiemes, Bettina Carvalho
and Rogerio Hamerschmidt

Abstract

Cochlear implant (CI) activation usually takes place at about 30 days postoperative (PO). In our service, CI surgery is performed with local anesthesia and sedation, so Activation is possible with the patient's cooperation, immediately after the CI surgery, still in the Operating Room (OR). The objective of this study was to provide the patient with hearing experience with the CI and to assess auditory perception immediately after surgery while still in the OR, and to compare Impedance Telemetry (IT), Neural Response Telemetry (NRT) and Comfort (C) level at two moments: in the OR and at the definitive Activation, approximately 30 days PO. Nine adults (12 ears) with acquired (post-lingual) deafness were included. Auditory perception was evaluated through Ling Sounds, musical instruments and clapping, presented in two different programming maps, elaborated using t-NRT, comparing between the two moments. We observed that while still in the OR, the patient can already present auditory detection and recognition responses. The values of impedance, t-NRT and "C" level on both dates differed with statistical significance. We concluded that it is possible to provide the patient with an auditory experience with the CI immediately after surgery, and that the auditory experience and the values of electrode IT, NRT and "C" level vary significantly between the two moments.

Keywords: cochlear implants, post-lingual hearing loss, neural response telemetry, impedance telemetry, hearing restoration

1. Introduction

Cochlear implants (CIs) are well established as a successful tool for treating deafness and providing access to sound in individuals with severe to profound bilateral hearing loss. The CI consists of an internal and an external unit. Among the internal unit components are: the receptor-stimulator, which includes the internal antenna, surgically placed next to the skull bone, behind the ear, under the skin, and the electrode array, which is positioned inside the cochlea. The external unit components are the microphone, speech processor and transmitting antenna. The CI partially replaces the functions of the cochlea, transforming sound energy into electrical signals. The auditory perception elicited by the CI depends on the amount of electrical current that passes through the system, and the amount of current needed for the sound stimulus to be perceived varies according to each individual and for each CI stimulation channel. The electrical stimulation parameters, therefore, must be individually adjusted to suit the needs of each patient.

The speech processor of the external unit is normally activated in the speech therapist's office, about 30–40 days after surgery, time necessary for adequate healing of the surgical wound. For this activation the speech processor is coupled to the computer software and, often using data obtained during the surgery, certain parameters are adjusted: stimulus current level, speed and pulse width. The adjustment process is called programming or "mapping," and the more accurate the mapping, the greater the potential for achieving adequate speech perception. This process takes time and must be performed regularly, as the use of the processor itself requires new adjustments, personalized programming for each individual, aiming at better hearing gain with increasingly clear, crisp and comfortable sound [1].

Mapping can be performed subjectively, through conditioning techniques and behavioral observation (clinical assessment) or objectively, through examinations. The common procedure in the programming of CI is the determination of the dynamic area for electrical stimulation. The dynamic area is the region between the amount of current that first induces an auditory sensation, that is, the threshold for electrical stimulation (T-level) and the maximum intensity sensation level that the patient will accept for electrical stimulation with comfort (C-level). The dynamic area is determined through psychophysical measures and the ease with which the speech therapist will obtain these levels varies according to a series of factors such as chronological age, mental conditions, time of deafness and other conditions of the patient's development. In young children or individuals with other associated impairments, obtaining the dynamic area is part of a long and complicated process, especially in the initial periods of CI use. The limited auditory experience that these individuals had before CI surgery, as well as the cognitive and linguistic immaturity to perform the necessary procedures, makes the answers obtained many times inconsistent. Although conditioning techniques and behavioral observation can be used to obtain T and C levels, unfortunately, for a part of the population, these values are not obtained reliably. As a result, these levels are often arbitrarily adjusted. On the other hand, objective measures may include electrically evoked brainstem potentials (EABR), stapedial reflex in response to electrical stimulation in the cochlea or standard measures of acoustic impedance. A more direct way of measuring cochlear nerve function is the Electrically Evoked Compound Action Potential (ECAP). ECAP reflects the synchronized firing of cochlear nerve fibers and is in many ways similar to wave I found in EABR, occurring at a latency of less than 0.5 ms. The Neural Response Telemetry (NRT) is a technique that allows direct measurement of ECAP in implanted patients [1]. *Behavioral assessment* includes musical instruments of low, medium and high timbres and with weak, medium and strong intensity. These instruments are: rattle, agogô, bell, drum, coco, rattle, castanets, ganzá, reco-reco, caxixi, xylophone, triangle, black black, accordion, whistle, cymbals. There are also methods that are attributed to evaluation, such as knocking on the door and clapping hands [2]. Composing the behavioral assessment, it is possible to make use of the "Sounds of LING" proposed by Daniel Ling, which incorporates phonemes of low, medium and high frequencies, which typically occur in speech [3], a behavioral assessment that tests the effectiveness of the cochlear implant. The concept behind Daniel Ling's Six Sound Test was to select familiar speech sounds that broadly represent the 250–8000 Hz speech spectrum. It is useful to address detection, discrimination and identification skills, but it is not a test of comprehension [4]. Auditory skills are: *detection*, which is the most basic level of sound perception, is awareness of the presence and absence of sound; *discrimination* is the ability to discriminate two or more stimuli, saying whether they are the same or different; the *recognition* skill that makes it possible to identify, classify and name what you have heard; and listening *comprehension* is considered the most complex, which allows the individual to understand the meaning of language in oral speech. Attention and memory processes permeate these skills and are essential for their development [4–6].

Objective assessment includes tests such as Impedance Telemetry that aims to assess the integrity and functionality of the electrode array and Neural Response Telemetry (NRT), which allows recording of the electrically evoked compound action potential (ECAP) of the distal portion of the auditory nerve, using the implant itself to elicit the stimulus and record the ECAP responses, evaluating the functional characteristics of ganglion cells and other neural structures [7, 8], which can be useful for programming the speech processor during the first postoperative adjustment [9] in patients who do not provide feedback, such as in young children. NRT is obtained in approximately 80% of the evaluated individuals and its technique can be a valuable tool in confirming the integrity of the internal device, in the objective determination of which electrodes can be included in a given map, the best stimulation speeds and speech coding strategies, as well as in the estimation of the dynamic area, with extreme clinical importance [10]. ECAP thresholds can be useful to predict the minimum and maximum levels that determine the dynamic area for electrical stimulation, these levels can be named and defined differently for the different brands of CI on the market. The dynamic area is the region between the amount of current that first induces the auditory sensation, that is, the threshold for electrical stimulation (T-level) and the maximum intensity sensation level that the patient will accept for electrical stimulation (C-level). This is done so that the CI is programmed within the loudness range which allows speech sounds and other sounds to be audible but not uncomfortable [11]. It is generally determined through psychophysical measurements, although objective or electrophysiological measurements of hearing can be used [12]. However the correlation between ECAP thresholds and psychophysical thresholds is affected by many factors, and analysis showed that there is only weak evidence to support the use of eCAP data for CI fitting purposes; and they are also an equally weak predictor for both T- and C-levels [13].

With the use of local anesthesia and sedation technique for CI surgery in our service [14], at the end of the surgery, still in the operating room, the patients are already awake and when the NRT is performed, they report listening to the stimuli that occur during the testing and sometimes may question if that is what they will hear after activating the CI.

With this report, we realized that it would be possible, even in the operating room, to activate the speech processor with patient cooperation, allowing the patient auditory perception immediately after surgery, still in the Operating Room. In this way we mapped the activation using the NRT thresholds to determine and test the dynamic field (T and C levels). After this activation, dressing of the wound was performed and the definitive activation was scheduled for about 30 days after this date, when adequate healing is achieved.

Therefore, the objective of this work was to carry out activation immediately after surgery while still in the Operating Room, providing the patient with an auditory experience with the CI, determining the dynamic field (T and C levels) and performing Impedance telemetry (IT), and Neural response telemetry (NRT) which is based on the measure of the Electric Compound Action Potential (ECAP) thresholds, using two different programming maps (Map 1 and 2) and comparing them at the moment of surgery and at the definitive Activation, 30 days later.

2. Materials and methods

This was a prospective analytical, longitudinal study, approved by the Institutional Review Board under number 12855619.9.0000.5529, carried out in nine adult patients (six unilateral and three bilateral cases, 12 ears total), all with acquired (post-lingual) hearing loss, who underwent CI surgery under local anesthesia and sedation according to our standard protocol published elsewhere 14 and who consented for the CI activation in the Operating Room (OR). Surgery was performed in the Operating Room of a tertiary hospital in the city of Curitiba, Parana, Brazil.

Patients either already were using Hearing Aids and underwent CI surgery (unilateral cases) or had a CI in one ear and underwent sequential CI surgery (bilateral cases). The sample included both sexes. Exclusion criteria were not consenting for the activation in the OR, not undergoing intraoperative NRT or failing (having no response) in assessment of impedance telemetry, or in obtaining intraoperative ECAP.

The CI model was CI24RE (CA) and CI422. Measurements were obtained during CI surgery through computer software NRT Custom Sound EP 3.2 (3.2.3855), connected to the portable programming unit and speech processor and the transmission antenna of the CI (software developed by Cochlear Corporation).

The NRT system allows pacing and recording on any pair of electrodes, in monopolar or bipolar modes. Normally, monopolar mode is used. The stimulation pulses are presented to a specific intracochlear electrode that has the MP1 extracochlear electrode as a reference, positioned below the temporal muscle flap. Another intracochlear electrode located in the vicinity is used as a recording electrode, having as reference another extracochlear electrode (MP2), located on the receptor-stimulator. Generally, the intracochlear electrode used for ECAP recording is located approximately 1.5 mm more apical (space of two electrodes) in relation to the position of the pacing electrode. For example, if the pacing electrode selected is 5, the recording electrode will be 7. The pair of active and reference electrodes used for pacing must be different from the pair of electrodes used for recording in order to reduce artifact. Electrodes with high impedance values or electrodes that are out of compliance should not be used for measurements.

Firstly, in the OR, Impedance Telemetry (IT) was performed to assess integrity and functionality of the electrodes. Impedances were measured on the 22 electrodes in monopolar MP1, monopolar MP2, monopolar MP1 + 2 and Common Ground (CG) modes. Values were considered normal when between 1.5 kΩ and 20 kΩ in MP1, MP2 and MP1 + 2 modes and between 0.7 kΩ and 20 kΩ in CG mode. Only electrodes that presented impedance within normal limits, according to software standards, were used for recording Neural Response Telemetry (NRT). Then, measurements of intraoperative t-NRT (NRT threshold) were performed in all electrodes, and we used the response in at least five electrodes for analysis, dividing the cochlea into four regions: electrodes 01 to 05, 06 to 10, 11 to 15 and 16 to 22. The current level (CL) in each electrode initiated at 150CL, with an interval of 6CL between one stimulus and the other, up to the maximum stimulation of 255CL or until reaching t-NRT. Interpulse interval was fixed at 500 μs, stimulation speed at 80 Hz in series of 25 μs per phase.

We used Cochlear Corporation Custom Sound EP software to obtain objective measurements of IT and NRT, and Custom Sound to assemble maps and perform Activation following surgery. With the Nucleus 5 - CP 810 processor, two maps were created with stimulation speed of 900 Hz, 8 maxima, volume 6, sensitivity 12, with different levels of "T" and "C":

- Map 1: Created with "C" levels by subtracting 10 current units from tNRT;
- Map 2: Created with "C" levels equal to tNRT.

And "T" levels were estimated at 40 current units below "C" level.

Afterwards, each patient was evaluated in the OR, with either map, by:

- Ling sounds (/a/, /i/, /u/, /m/, /s/, /sh/);
- Instrumental sounds: bell rattle (2KHz to 6KHz), coconut shells (600 Hz to 3KHz), bell (4KHz to 8KHz) and drum (250 Hz to 600 Hz) (**Figure 1**);
- Claps (one or two claps).

Presentations were performed in a closed set, the patient being informed about which sounds would be presented: Ling Sounds, musical instruments or clapping. All were performed approximately 60 cm from the speech processor. The patient was still lying on the surgical table. Responses were observed and noted. The analysis of the

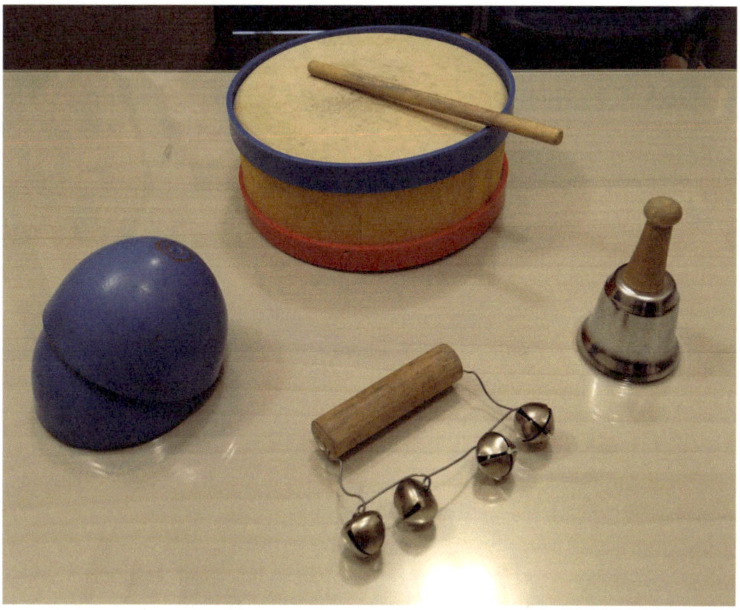

Figure 1.
Instruments sounds used: Bell rattle, coconut shells, bell and drum.

auditory perception responses, immediately after surgery, in the two different maps tested, was done by observational analysis. The behavioral tests were evaluated based on the auditory skills: detection, discrimination and recognition.

The second assessment was done at the day of definite activation, 30 days postop, with IT and NRT.

Results were described as mean, standard deviation (SD), median, minimum and maximum. To compare NRT and IT between the two evaluation moments, Student's t test was used for paired samples. The normality condition was evaluated by the Shapiro-Wilk test. Values of $p < 0.05$ were considered of statistical significance. Data were analyzed using the computer program Stata/SE v.14.1. StataCorpLP, USA. Detection, recognition and non-detection to sound were considered for the observational analysis of responses to Ling Sounds, instrumental and clapping sounds.

3. Results

The analysis performed was based on data from 12 ears of nine patients (six unilateral and three bilateral cases). The CI electrode bundle CI24RE (CA) was used for 10 ears and two ears with CI422. Based on the presented tNRT, Maps 1 and 2 were tested. We based the analysis in that sound detection precedes auditory recognition, so all percentage calculations were based on the total detection and recognition being 100%, and from this we calculated the percentage of recognition.

For the detection, non-detection and recognition of Ling Sounds in the 12 ears, we found that with Map 1: the 12 ears detected the phoneme /a/, but only 3 ears recognized it, the 12 ears detected /i/, but only 2 recognized it, 11 detected /u/, 3 recognized it, 11 detected /m/, 12 detected /sh/ and one recognized it, 12 detected /s/. With Map 2, for the phoneme /a/ 12 detected and 5 recognized it, for /i/ 12 detected and 2 recognized it, for /u/ 12 detected and 6 recognized it, for /m/ 12 detected and 2 recognized it, for /sh/ 12 detected and 4 recognized it, and for /s/ 12 detected and 1 recognized it. Based on these data we can say that we obtained 12.85% of recognition of LING sounds for Map 1 and 27.77% with Map 2.

For the detection, non-detection and auditory recognition of musical instruments with Map 1, there was detection of the bell rattle, coconut shells, bell and drum for the 12 ears, 3 of which recognized the bell and 3 recognized the drum. As for Map 2, there was detection of the bell rattle for 11 ears, for the other instruments there was detection with the 12 ears, and 2 ears recognized the bell, and 3 the drum. Therefore, it was possible to observe 25% of recognition of the bell and drum for Map 1 and 16.66% of recognition for the bell and 25% for the drum with Map 2.

For the detection, non-detection and recognition of one or two claps we verified that palms were possible to be detected and recognized. With Map 1 we found 41.66% of recognition for one or two claps and with Map 2 the recognition was 33.33%. With both Map 1 and Map 2, some patients reported detecting and discriminating the sound, but they did not recognize it (they did not know what they were hearing). They detected but made mismatches between Ling Sounds, between the instruments, and named instruments such as "hiss," "beat," "a thin sound," or "papapa." With Map 1, the rattle (that was not presented) was also mentioned, and one patient reported hearing well and one reported hearing it low. With Map 2, three patients reported being too loud, one patient reported discriminating between low and high sounds. All these responses were considered detection. Only those who recognized the sound being presented were considered recognition. Results were similar for all patients in both maps, although discomfort was reported with Map 2 (stronger) by three patients.

Regarding tNRT, **Table 1** presents descriptive statistics of tNRT in the operating room and on activation and the mean difference between tNRT in the two situations.

Based on **Table 1**, we can see that there was a statistically significant difference between tNRT obtained in the OR and on the day of definitive activation for electrodes 1, 6, 11 and 16, only not for electrode 22 (but p value suggests that there is a tendency for a statistically significant difference).

Table 2 shows descriptive statistics of tNRT in the operating room and the measurements of "C" level informed by the patient on the day of activation and the mean difference between them. There was a statistical difference between tNRT measurement performed in the OR and the measurement of the "C" level informed by the patient on the day of activation as a comfort level. We can observe that the values of the "average and median" of the current levels for each electrode decrease between one situation and another.

We can see clearly how in the three situations (*tNRT on the day of surgery, tNRT on the day of definitive activation and "C" level* on the day of activation) *current level decreases*.

Table 3 presents descriptive statistics of IT in the OR and at activation 30 days later and the average difference between IT in the two situations. There was a statistically significant difference between the two moments. *It is clear how Impedance values increased consecutively*.

Electrode	Variable	Mean ± SD	Median (min-max)	Mean reduction (OR – activation)	p*
Electrode 1	tNRT OR	180.7 ± 19.6	182.5 (145–205)	14.8	<0.001
	tNRT activation	165.8 ± 21.6	169.5 (126–191)		
Electrode 6	tNRT OR	187.3 ± 14.9	184.5 (162–215)	15.2	<0.001
	tNRT activation	172.1 ± 10.8	173 (155–194)		
Electrode 11	tNRT OR	193.3 ± 16.5	199,5 (165–217)	13.1	0.015
	tNRT activation	180.3 ± 20.7	189 (134–203)		
Electrode 16	tNRT OR	184.1 ± 20.4	185 (141–220)	11.2	0.016
	tNRT activation	172.9 ± 16.4	176 (135–191)		
Electrode 22	tNRT OR	170.9 ± 19.2	175 (140–204)	13.8	0.091
(n = 11)	tNRT activation	157.1 ± 18.6	154 (129–190)		

*OR = operating room, activation = activation day; min-max = minimum and maximum values; SD = standard deviation. *Student's t test for paired samples, p < 0.05.*

Table 1.
Comparison between tNRT values: in the operating room (OR) and at the activation day (after 30 days).

Electrode	Variable	Mean ± SD	Median (min-max)	Mean reduction (OR – "C")	p*
Electrode 1	tNRT OR	180.7 ± 19.6	182.5 (145–205)	40.7	<0.001
	"C" level activation	139.9 ± 21.1	140 (102–175)		
Electrode 6	tNRT OR	187.3 ± 14.9	184.5 (162–215)	43.5	<0.001
	"C" level activation	143.8 + 14.1	146 (122–162)		
Electrode 11	tNRT OR	193.3 ± 16.5	199.5 (165–217)	46.4	<0.001
	"C" level activation	146.9 ± 12.7	147.5 (130–165)		
Electrode 16	tNRT OR	184.1 ± 20.4	185 (141–220)	38.2	<0.001
	"C" level activation	145.8 ± 12.3	147 (126–165)		
Electrode 22	tNRT OR	170.9 ± 19.2	175 (140–204)	29.4	0.001
(n = 11)	"C" level activation	141.5 ± 11.4	138 (127–165)		

*OR = operating room, activation = activation day; min-max = minimum and maximum values; SD = standard deviation. *Student's t test for paired samples, $p < 0.05$.*

Table 2.
Comparison between tNRT in the operating room (OR) and the "C" level assessment (activation with responses) (after 30 days).

4. Discussion

We observed that in our CI patients because of the local anesthesia and sedation technique [14] it was possible to perform CI activation at the immediate period of surgery, while still in the Operating Room (OR). We also found that we can use tNRT as a "C" level of stimulation.

In our study, we found that there was a statistically significant difference in telemetry (both IT and tNRT comparing OR day and day of activation), in that IT increased after surgery, and tNRT and C level decreased after surgery; in the OR there was detection in behavioral tests with Ling Sounds, musical instruments and clapping, but discomfort to the sound was also reported. Due to this discomfort, we therefore suggest using a lower current level for activation than the one found on tNRT at the day of surgery.

Lai et al. [15] showed that intraoperative NRT data were generally stable enough to be used to assist in initial speech processor mappings, and it was not possible to predict changes in the map's subjective threshold or comfortable loudness levels based on changes observed in the NRT data. In our study, we warn that this should be done with caution, because there was a statistically significant difference when comparing tNRT responses on the day of surgery with the measurement of "C" level (comfort

Electrode	Variable	Mean ± SD	Median (min-max)	Mean increase (ativ – CC)	p*
Electrode 1	IT OR	57 ± 1.5	5.7 (3.9–8.7)	8.3	<0.001
	IT activation	13.9 ± 2.2	14 (9.6–17)		
Electrode 6	IT OR	5.1 ± 2.1	5.1 (2.5–9.7)	7.9	<0.001
	IT activation	13 ± 2.2	13.1 (7.7–15.7)		
Electrode 11	IT OR	5.6 ± 2.2	5.2 (2.9–10.9)	6.2	<0.001
	IT activation	11.8 ± 2	12.2 (7.6–13.8)		
Electrode 16	IT OR	5.8 ± 2.0	5 (3.6–10.1)	5.6	<0.001
	IT activation	11.4 ± 2.8	12.3 (6.6–15.1)		
Electrode 22	IT OR	6.3 ± 2.6	5.3 (3.2–10.6)	5.4	<0.001
	IT activation	11.8 ± 3.3	12 (4.4–16.8)		

*OR = operating room, activation = activation day; min-max = minimum and maximum values; SD = standard deviation. *Student's t test for paired samples, $p < 0.05$.*

Table 3.
Comparison between electrode impedance telemetry (IT) in the operating room (OR) and in the activation day (after 30 days).

threshold) at the day of activation. These values decreased, tNRT in OR was higher than tNRT on the day of definitive activation, and this in turn was higher than the "C" level measured on the day of definitive activation. Unlike tNRT, we observed that Impedance values increased from the day of surgery to the day of activation, but it should be noted that IT was the first procedure performed and the stimulation current had still passed. Often, when we perform CI activation in young children, who do not cooperate or who do not allow tNRT to be performed, we use tNRT performed in the OR as basis for building the activation map. It is important to know, although it is information given by an adult, how much the tNRT data performed on the day of surgery can help but also be uncomfortable in the listening experience. In this study, we observed that the map with the "C" level at the tNRT threshold, although considered uncomfortable by two patients, because it was higher, allowed the detection of Ling Sounds, clapping and the detection of instruments only reporting whether bass or treble. Of course, with children we should rely much more on observing behavioral responses and make use of other objective measures such as the investigation of the electrically evoked stapedial reflex threshold [16]. It is important to emphasize that when programming levels are determined based on ECAP thresholds, the stimulation can be uncomfortably high, particularly in the basal electrodes [17–19]. We could observe that there was a decrease of about 40cu for the basal electrodes between the ECAP thresholds (tNRT) on the day of surgery (OR) and the "C" level reported by the patient at the Activation day.

More research is needed to affirm whether the eCAP can be used to predict current levels of individual CI recipients at the day of activation [13]. But our findings can be of help.

Behavioral measures, even if minimally observable, are important for CI programming. Objective electrophysiological measurements help predict behavioral levels, but these alone cannot replace the accuracy of a behavioral map [20]. Research has revealed a stronger correlation between ECAP threshold and "C" level than between ECAP threshold and "T" level [21]. We believe that our patients found it easy to detect the sound and even to recognize it, because they had all post-lingual hearing loss and already wore a CI in one ear or hearing aids. *We have previously studied pre- and post-lingual differences in programming elsewhere* [22]. It was possible to observe with Map 2, level "C" at the NRT threshold, a higher percentage of detection and recognition of Ling sounds when compared to Map 1. Regarding the instruments, we used instruments with different sound spectrum: for the bell rattle, detection was considered the fact that they identified the sound and reported being strong or weak and being high or low, we could observe that only for one ear with Map 2 the bell rattle was not detected.

In this research, it was possible to observe that even immediately after the insertion of the electrode bundle in the cochlea, while still in the OR, the patient can already present auditory detection and recognition responses with both objective and behavioral measures. We believe in the importance of activation as early as possible, but we agree that the healing period must be respected. This auditory experience may make them calmer and hopeful to wait for the definitive Activation date in 30 days and this observation may also help in the programming of the CI.

5. Conclusion

This chapter shows that CI activation in the Operating Room, immediately after surgery with local anesthesia and sedation, is possible. We could provide the patient with a hearing experience with the CI while still in the OR with auditory detection and auditory discrimination of different types of stimuli, but with poor recognition. Maps with higher current offer better results, but also provide auditory discomfort. Impedance telemetry values increased from the day of surgery to the day of definitive activation, at 30 days, and Neural Response Telemetry values decreased for the same period, and both were statistically significant.

Conflicts of interest

None to declare.

Author details

Gislaine Richter Minhoto Wiemes[1], Nicole Richter Minhoto Wiemes[1],
Bettina Carvalho[1,2]* and Rogerio Hamerschmidt[1,2]

1 Hospital Paranaense de Otorrinolaringologia, Curitiba, Pr, Brazil

2 Complexo Hospital de Clínicas da UFPR, Curitiba, Pr, Brazil

*Address all correspondence to: bettinacarvalho@yahoo.com.br

References

[1] Ferrari D, Sameshima K, Costa Filho O, Bevilacqua MC. Neural response telemetry on the nucleus 24 multichannel cochlear implant system: Literature review. Revista Brasileira de Oto-Rino-Laringologia. 2004;**70**(1):112-118

[2] Souza MF, Corazza MC, Quintilio R. Acoustic analysis of musical instruments used for child audiology evaluation. Rev Inic Cient e Ext. 2018;**1**(Esp.3):272-282

[3] Ling D. Foundations of Spoken Language for the Hearing-Impaired Child. Washington, DC: Alexander Graham Bell Association for the Deaf; 1989

[4] Smiley DF, Martin PF, Lance DM. Using the Ling 6-sound test everyday [Internet]. Audiology Online 2004. Available from: https://www.audiologyonline.com/articles/using-ling-6-sound-test-1087

[5] Quique Y. Métodos unisensoriales para la rehabilitación de la persona con implante coclear y métodos musicoterapéuticos como nueva herramienta de intervención. Rev Otorrinolaringol Cir Cabeza Cuello. 2013;**73**:94-108

[6] Comerlatto MPS. Habilidades auditivas e de linguagem de crianças usuários de implante coclear análise dos marcadores clínicos de desenvolvimento. Mariane Perin de Silva Comerlato - São Paulo. Tese (doutorado)- Faculdade de Medicina da Universidade de São Paulo: 2015

[7] Abbas PJ, Brown CJ, Shallop JK, Firszt JB, Hughes ML, Hong SH, et al. Summary of results using the nucleus CI24M implant to record the electrically evoked compound action potential. Ear and Hearing. 1999;**20**(1):45-49

[8] Guedes MC, Weber R, Goffi-Gomez MV, Brito Neto RV, Peralta CG, Bento RF. Telemetria de resposta neural intraoperatória em usuários de implante coclear. Revista Brasileira de Oto-Rino-Laringologia. 2005;**71**(5):660-667

[9] Grolman W, Maat A, Verdam F, Simis Y, Carelsen B, Freling N, et al. Spread of excitation measurements for the detection of electrode Array Foldovers: A prospective study comparing 3-dimensional rotational X-ray and intraoperative spread of excitation measurements. Otology & Neurotology. 2009;**30**(2):27-33

[10] Shallop JK, Facer GW, Peterson A. Neural response telemetry with the nucleus CI24M Cochlear implant. The Laryngoscope. 1999;**109**(11):1755-1759

[11] Roberts S. Speech-processor fitting for cochlear implants. In: Cooper H, editor. Cochlear Implants: A Practical Guide. London: Whurr Publishers; 1991. pp. 201-218

[12] Shapiro W. Device programming. In: Waltzman SB, Cohen NL, editors. Cochlear Implants. New York: Thieme; 2000. pp. 185-198

[13] Ji F, Liu K, Yang S. Clinical application of electrically evoked compound action potentials. Journal of Otology. 2014;**9**:117-121

[14] Hamerschmidt R, Moreira AT, Wiemes GR, Tenório S, Tâmbara EM. Cochlear implant surgery with local anaesthesia and sedation: Comparison with general anaesthesia. Otology & Neurotology. 2013;**34**(1):75-78

[15] Lai WK, Aksit M, Akdas F, Diller N. Longitudinal behaviour of

neural response telemetry (NRT) data and clinical implications. International Journal of Audiology. 2004;**43**(5):252-263

[16] Andrade KC, Leal MC, Muniz LF, Menezes PL, Albuquerque KM, Carnaúba AT. The importance of electrically evoked stapedial reflex in cochlear implant. Brazilian Journal of Otorhinolaryngology. 2014;**80**(1):68-77

[17] Eisen MD, Franck KH. Electrically evoked compound action potential amplitude growth functions and HiResolution programming levels in paediatric CII implant subjects. Ear and Hearing. 2004;**25**(6):528e538

[18] Han DM, Chen XQ, Zhao XT, Kong Y, Li YX, Liu S. Comparisons between neural response imaging thresholds, electrically evoked auditory reflex thresholds and most comfortable loudness levels in CII bionic ear users with HiResolution sound processing strategies. Acta Oto-Laryngologica. 2005;**125**(7):732e735

[19] Jeon EK, Brown CJ, Etler CP, O'Brien S, Chiou LK, Abbas PJ. Comparison of electrically evoked compound action potential thresholds and loudness estimates for the stimuli used to program the advanced bionics cochlear implant. Journal of the American Academy of Audiology. 2010;**21**(1):16e27

[20] Raghunandhan S, Ravikumar A, Kameswaran M, Mandke K, Ranjith R. Electrophysiological correlates of behavioural comfort levels in Cochlear Implantees: A prospective study. Indian Journal of Otolaryngology Head and Neck Surgery. 2015;**67**(3):210-222

[21] Holstad BA, Sonneveldt VG, Fears BT, Davidson LS, Aaron RJ, Richter M, et al. Relation of electrically evoked compound action potential thresholds to behavioural T- and C-levels in children with cochlear implants. Ear and Hearing. 2009;**30**(1):115e127

[22] Carvalho B, Wiemes GRM, Patrial Netto L, Hamerschmidt R. Neural recovery function of the auditory nerve in Cochlear implant surgery: Comparison between Prelingual and Postlingual patients. International Archeological Otorhinolaryngology. 2020;**24**(4):e444-e449

Chapter 8

Static Posturography with Nintendo Balance Board in Children after Cochlear Implantation

Maksym Situkho, Viktor Lutsenko, Yevhen Antonov and Viliam Dolinay

Abstract

Human balance is essential for maintaining stable posture and safe mobility. Balance relies on the integration of various sensory and motor systems, including the audiovestibular, visual, and proprioceptive systems. Cochlear implantation can potentially affect the peripheral vestibular system, leading to balance disturbances. We studied postural balance in children after cochlear implantation (CI) using the Nintendo Wii Balance Board (WBB) with Wii Posturografie software. Balance was assessed in 77 children (14 with CI, 25 with sensorineural deafness, and 38 controls). Children under 8 years old after CI showed significant differences in postural balance compared to controls, while those over 8 years old did not differ significantly. The WBB with Wii Posturografie proves effective for evaluating postural balance in children. Understanding postural changes in CI recipients can aid in optimizing auditory rehabilitation and enhancing overall outcomes. Further long-term investigations are needed.

Keywords: cochlear implantation, postural balance, static posturography, Nintendo Wii Balance Board, children

1. Introduction

Human balance is a multidimensional concept, referring to the ability of a person to avoid falling. It can be characterized as the potential of the body to maintain a stable posture for maximum time with minimal body sway. The integration and coordination of various body systems, including the audiovestibular, visual, and motor systems, as well as higher-level premotor systems, contribute to achieving balance. The central nervous system interprets information from sensory systems and produces a response to activate postural muscular synergies. These synergies are responsible for proper head, eye, and body movements to maintain posture [1].

Balance maintenance involves holding, attaining, or restoring the projection of a center of pressure (COP) relative to the support base, or generally within the limit of stability. The limit of stability is the maximum deviation of the body that a person can arbitrarily withstand in any direction without falling or having to take a step [2].

The functions of the balance system include [3]:

1. Maintaining a certain postural position, such as sitting or standing.

2. Promoting voluntary movements such as transitional movements between postures.

3. Reactions that restore equilibrium after sudden external stimuli such as a trip, a slip, or a push.

Balance control is essential not only to maintain postural stability but also to ensure safe mobility in everyday life, such as performing manual tasks while standing, lifting from a chair, walking, and turning.

The balance is usually tested on a force platform in a laboratory setting. Force platforms are commonly found in research laboratories, physiotherapy, and audiology departments because they can be used to identify most types of balance disorders, are available commercially, and have normative data associated with them [4].

During the study, the body sway data, a factor directly related to the balance, is obtained by recording the force vector applied by the body to the plane of the platform. The data obtained allow us to describe the body sway using several quantitative indicators accurately.

There are some important limitations. Testing on the force platform is a time-consuming procedure, the platform itself requires installation under the floor, which restricts its mobility and significantly increases the overall cost of the equipment. Thus, the classical force platform is difficult to use in conventional clinical practice.

The Wii Balance Board (WBB) device (Nintendo, Kyoto, Japan) is relatively inexpensive and available almost anywhere in the world, but it is potentially effective to perform an instrumental balance assessment in limited time and space clinical settings. This device resembles a typical force platform (**Figure 1**) and is a clinically useful tool for assessing balance [5].

Scientists from several countries are using WBB with adapted or custom software, such as LabView (National Instruments, Austin, TX, USA), Balancia (Mintosys, Seoul, Korea), Wii Posturografie (Tomas Bata University, Zlin, Chech Republic) that communicates with WBB via Bluetooth to evaluate differences with laboratory-level force platforms [5–7]. WBB demonstrated excellent concurrent validity in comparison with force platforms to quantify static balance in healthy adults (ICC 0.77 to >0.99) and in patients with Parkinson's disease (ICC = 0.92–0.98) after stroke (ICC = 0.82–0.98) [8, 9].

Various pathologies such as neurological disorders, sensory deficits, or muscle weakness can cause balance disorders.

Deafness is one of the most severe sensory deficits for an individual and for society as a whole. At the same time, vestibular dysfunction is often detected in children with congenital hearing defects. According to Jacot (2008), the vestibular function was symmetrically impaired on both sides in 18.6%, asymmetrically impaired in 32.6%, and was normal only in 37.2% of cases among patients with deafness [8].

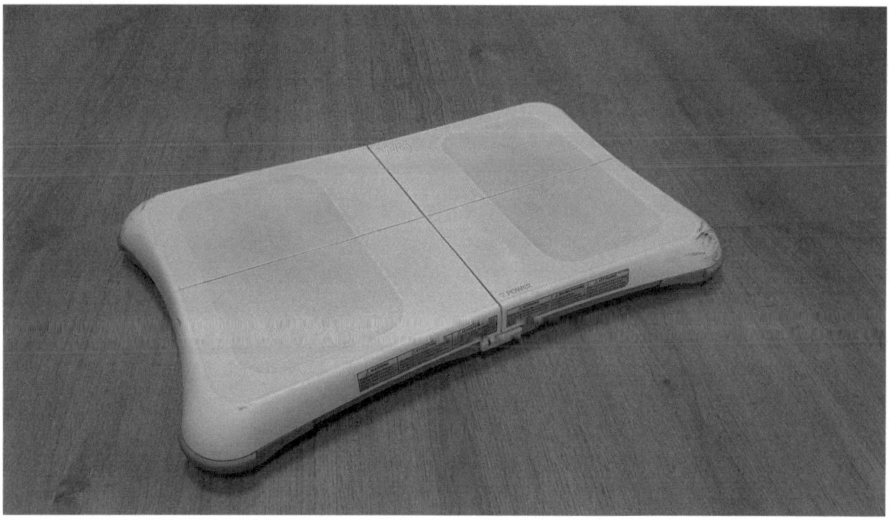

Figure 1.
Wii balance board platform.

Cochlear implantation (CI) is a state-of-the-art and the most effective method of deafness rehabilitation. More than one million patients worldwide are already users of cochlear implants [9].

Both intraoperatively and in the postoperative period of cochlear implantation, a negative effect on the peripheral part of the vestibular analyzer is possible due to several mechanisms:

- direct traumatization of the vestibule with an active electrode [10];
- intraoperative loss of perilymph [11];
- acute serous labyrinthitis after cochleostomy [12];
- the reaction of the labyrinth to a foreign body [13];
- endolymphatic hydrops [14];
- electrical stimulation of the labyrinth [15].

The following manifestations of vestibular dysfunction after exposure to the above factors have been described [11, 12, 16]:

- worsening of the existing vestibular dysfunction;
- the onset of vestibular dysfunction after CI;
- slowing down the development of motor skills;
- disequilibrium;
- dizziness caused by sound.

Given the critical social impact of CI, especially in children, all of these potential negative effects should be investigated in great detail. Despite a large number of clinical trials performed in the world and in Ukraine, the state of postural balance in patients in the long-term period has not been studied enough. This is due to the low motivation of the parents of implanted children to undergo additional examinations, especially in the absence of complaints in the child, as well as the unavailability of equipment for the study of balance in routine clinical practice.

Purpose of the study: To study the indicators of postural balance in children after cochlear implantation.

An observational cohort study included 38 children with normal hearing and no vestibular complaints, 25 children with sensorineural deafness (SND), and 14 children after unilateral cochlear implantation. The age of the children ranged from 2.8 to 17.9 years. The mean time after implantation was 3.2 years.

Static balance was assessed using the Nintendo Wii Balance Board (Nintendo, Kyoto, Japan) connected via Bluetooth to a Dell 3550 laptop (Dell Inc., Round Rock, USA). WBB accuracy in weight measurement was assessed by the state metrological enterprise "Ukrmetrteststandart". Postural balance indicators were recorded using the Wii Posturografie software developed at the Department of Applied Informatics at Tomas Bata University (Zlín, Czech Republic) (**Figure 2**).

The study was conducted in a quiet medical office, the patient stood barefoot on the platform in a position with heels together, feet apart at an angle of 45°. The child was given up 30 s to adapt, then the balance indicators were recorded in a position with open eyes for 20 s. After that, the child was asked to close his eyes, after adaptation, the balance indicators were recorded in the position with eyes closed for the next 20 s [17]. All indicators in children after cochlear implantation were recorded with the processor turned on.

The following postural balance parameters were recorded: Way, Area, Lateral, Anterior-Posterior (AP), and AP/Lateral in the position with gaze fixation (Opened) and with eyes closed (Closed). The following indicators were calculated: Romberg Way, Romberg Area [18]. See **Table 1a** (**Appendix**) for the list of technical terms.

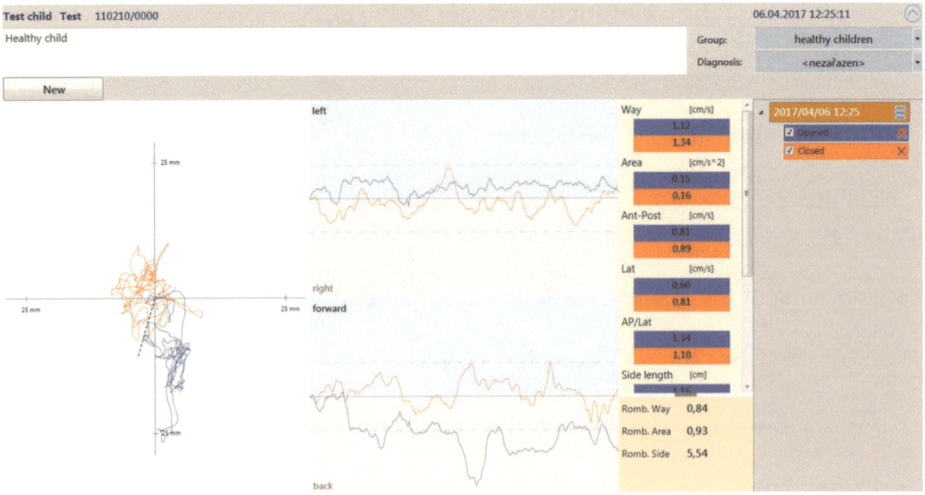

Figure 2.
Wii posturography software interface.

The following indicators are considered the most critical balance parameters:

The Way parameter (cm/s) describes the path of movement of the COP. Since the study time is set to a constant number, this parameter is characterized as the speed of COP.

$$M_i = \sqrt{(x_{i+1} - x_i)_2 + (y_{i+1} - y_i)^2}$$
$$W = \frac{T^{-1}}{n} \sum_{i=1}^{n} M_i [mm/s], \quad (1)$$

Where:

Me – a separate element of the path calculation

T – study period

x,y – coordinates of COP

n – number of measurements

The Area parameter (cm^2/s) marks the area and describes the variations in COP during the study.

$$N_i = \frac{\left|(y_{i+1} - y_0) * (x_i - x_o) - (y_i - y_o) * (x_{i+1} - x_0)\right|}{2}$$

$$A = \frac{1}{t} \sum_{i=1}^{n-1} N_i \left[\mathrm{mm}^2/s\right], \quad (2)$$

Where:

N_i – a separate element of the area calculation,

t – study duration [s],

x_O and y_O - average values of the coordinates of the center of gravity.

The AP parameter is the resulting anteroposterior center of gravity vector (the length of the anteroposterior COP shifts during the study).

$$sum = \sum_{i=1} (y_i - y_{i-1})$$
$$Ant\text{-}Post = sum/t, \quad (3)$$

Where:

t – study duration [ms],

y – the center of coordinates of COP.

The parameter Lateral (cm/s) is the resulting amplitude vector of the lateral displacements of the center of gravity (the length of the lateral displacements of the center of gravity during the study).

$$sum = \sum_{i=1} (x_i - x_{i-1})$$
$$Lateral = sum/t \quad (4)$$

Where:

t – study duration [ms],

x – the center of coordinates of the center of gravity.

The AP/Lateral parameter is the ratio of the anterior–posterior and lateral balance components of the subject. It reflects the general dominance of the direction of the gravitational amplitude.

$$\frac{AP}{Lateral} = \frac{Ant - Post}{Lateral} \tag{5}$$

All parameters were recorded in two positions: with eyes open (opened) with gaze fixed on a still image and in a state with eyes closed (closed). In the first position, the vestibular system, visual posture control, and the proprioceptive system are involved in maintaining balance. In the second position, the participation of visual control in maintaining postural balance is excluded.

The Romberg Way parameter is the ratio of the Way values obtained in the study with the patient's eyes open and closed.

$$Romberg\ Way = \frac{Way_{closed}}{Way_{opened}} \tag{6}$$

The Romberg Area parameter is the ratio of the Area values obtained in the study with the patient's eyes open and closed.

$$Romberg\ Area = \frac{Area_{close}}{Area_{opened}} \tag{7}$$

The Romberg Way and Romberg Area parameters demonstrate the role of visual control in maintaining postural balance.

Statistical processing included testing the hypothesis that the sample distribution corresponds to a normal (Gaussian) distribution using the Kolmogorov–Smirnov and Shapiro–Wilk tests. The null hypothesis of the absence of differences between the samples in multiple comparisons was tested using the nonparametric Kruskal–Wallace test. The Spearman correlation coefficient was used to determine the relationship between individual indicators.

Differences between samples were considered statistically significant at a significance level p (probability of erroneously rejecting the null hypothesis) less than 0.05. Data analysis was carried out using the MedCalc statistical software (MedCalc Software Ltd., Ostend, Belgium). Graphs and figures showing the differences between the indicators were obtained using the MedCalc software.

2. Results and discussion

Based on the literature data [19, 20], we conducted a correlation analysis of the relationship between postural balance indicators and age in children with normal hearing (**Figure 3**). We recorded a trend toward a significant decrease in the values of indicators until the age of 8 years. With increasing age, the balance indicators stabilized or had a slight tendency to decrease. As a result of the subsequent analysis, we obtained significant differences in the values of the postural balance parameters Way, Area, and AP recorded in the position with eyes closed and the values of the AP parameter recorded with eyes open in children in groups younger than and older than 8 years (**Table 1**).

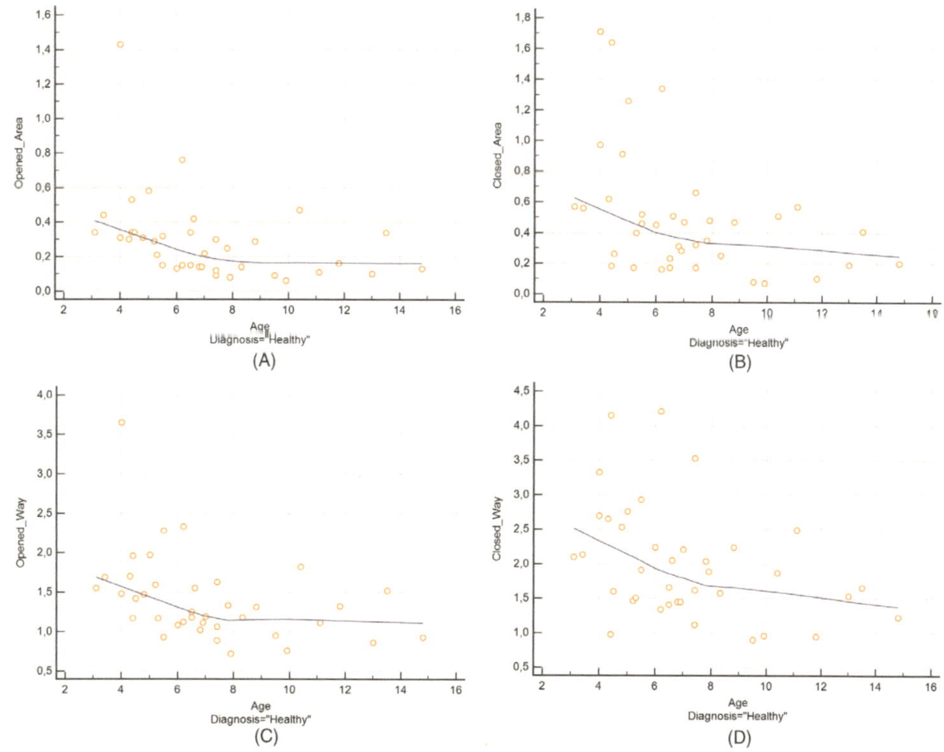

Figure 3.
Correlation analysis of postural balance parameters in children with normal hearing depending on their age. A. Parameter Area with opened eyes. B. Parameter Area with closed eyes. C. Parameter Way with opened eyes. D. Parameter Way with closed eyes.

	Under 8 years old Median (95% CI)		Over 8 years old Median (95% CI)	
	Eyes opened	**Eyes closed**	**Eyes opened**	**Eyes closed**
Way, cm/s	1.38 (1.12–1.66)	2.05 (1.49–2.68)	1.15 (0.93–1.32)	1.56 (0.96–1.87)*
Area, cm/s^2	0.30 (0.15–0.34)	0.47 (0.27–0.64)	0.13 (0.10–0.29)*	0.23 (0.10–0.47)*
AP, cm/s	0.91 (0.78–1.17)	1.56 (1.09–1.87)	0.75 (0.64–0.92)	1.03 (0.71–1.22)*
Lateral, cm/sec	0.83 (0.66–1.02)	1.05 (0.8–1.52)	0.71 (0.54–0.78)	0.77 (0.55–1.25)
AP/Lateral	1.15 (0.95–1.29)	1.35 (1.16–1.54)	1.16 (1.03–1.23)	1.27 (0.98–1.54)

*Note: CI, confidence interval; *, the difference between indicators in groups under 8 and over 8 years old is statistically significant ($p < 0.05$).*

Table 1.
Postural balance parameters in normally hearing children.

In this work, we divided all groups of children (control, CIS, after CT) into 2 age subgroups: up to eight and after eight full years.

The results obtained are shown in **Tables 2–4**.

2.1 Parameter way

In the position with open eyes (Opened) in children under 8 years of age, the Way parameter significantly differed from the control both in the group of children with

Parameter	Median (95% CI)					
	Eyes opened			Eyes closed		
	Normal hearing	SND	Cochlear implantation	Normal hearing	SND	Cochlear implantation
Way, cm/s	1.38 (1.12–1.66)	2.50 (1.44–3.03)*	2.70 (1.98–4.65)*	2.05 (1.49–2.68)	2.59 (1.88–4.63)	3.78 (2.96–3.87)*
Area, cm/s^2	0.30 (0.15–0.34)	0.57 (0.30–1.44)*	0.88 (0.43–2.72)*	0.47 (0.27–0.64)	0.70 (0.46–1.65)*	1.45 (0.74–1.72)*
AP, cm/s	0.91 (0.78–1.17)	1.56 (0.99–2.12)*	2.04 (1.32–2.45)*	1.56 (1.09–1.87)	1.88 (1.37–3.19)*	2.71 (2.04–2.91)*
Lateral, cm/sec	0.83 (0.66–1.02)	1.56 (0.86–1.78)*	1.62 (0.90–3.39)*	1.05 (0.8–1.52)	1.43 (1.03–2.30)	1.99 (1.13–2.13)*
AP/Lateral	1.15 (0.95–1.29)	1.16 (1.04–1.25)	1.17 (0.79–1.48)	1.35 (1.16–1.54)	1.36 (1.16–1.57)	1.37 (1.36–1.80)

*Note: CI, confidence interval; *, a significant difference was revealed between the parameter values in comparison with children with normal hearing ($p < 0.05$).*

Table 2.
Postural balance parameters in children under 8 years old.

Parameter	Median (95% CI)					
	Eyes opened			Eyes closed		
	Normal hearing	SND	Cochlear implantation	Normal hearing	SND	Cochlear implantation
Way, cm/s	1.15 (0.93–1.32)	1.03 (0.76–1.33)	0.89 (0.78–0.96)	1.56 (0.96–1.87)	1.59 (1.15–2.09)	1.45 (1.16–2.12)
Area, cm/s^2	0.14 (0.10–0.29)	0.17 (0.09–0.26)	0.14 (0.07–0.20)	0.23 (0.10–0.47)	0.27 (0.17–0.68)	0.25 (0.21–0.51)
AP, cm/s	0.75 (0.64–0.92)	0.73 (0.48–0.88)	0.62 (0.54–0.67)	1.03 (0.71–1.22)	1.21 (0.81–1.43)	0.96 (0.75–1.52)
Lateral, cm/sec	0.71 (0.54–0.78)	0.62 (0.46–0.82)	0.55 (0.44–0.57)	0.77 (0.55–1.25)	0.87 (0.70–1.19)	0.85 (0.65–1.00)
AP/Lateral	1.16 (1.03–1.23)	1.08 (1.05–1.36)	1.20 (1.10–1.33)	1.27 (0.98–1.54)	1.32 (1.20–1.61)	1.08 (1.01–2.14)

Note: CI, confidence interval.

Table 3.
Postural balance parameters in children over 8 years old.

	Under 8 years old Median (95% CI)			Over 8 years old Median (95% CI)		
	Normal hearing	**SND**	**Cochlear implantation**	**Normal hearing**	**SND**	**Cochlear implantation**
Romberg Way	0.75 (0.55–0.82)	0.81 (0.76–0.95)	0.69 (0.59–1.65)	0.78 (0.58–0.97)	0.60 (0.46–0.81)	0.52 (0.45–0.76)
Romberg Area	0.59 (0.40–0.86)	0.69 (0.63–1.06)	0.72 (0.50–2.30)	0.74 (0.56–0.92)	0.53 (0.23–0.59)	0.34 (0.29–0.72)

Note: CI, confidence interval.

Table 4.
Parameters Romberg way and Romberg area.

SND and in the group of children after CI (p = 0.000260), and there was no significant difference between the SND and CI groups. At the same time, in children older than 8 years, there was no significant difference in the Way parameters between the groups.

In the position with eyes closed (Closed) in children under 8 years of age, the Way parameter was statistically significantly higher only in the CI group (p = 0.011218), in the control group and CIS there was no statistically significant difference.

In children older than 8 years, there was no statistically significant difference between the groups either in the position with eyes open (p = 0.225619) or in the position with eyes closed (p = 0.857089).

2.2 Parameter area

In the position with open eyes (Opened) in children under 8 years old, the Area parameter significantly differed from the control both in the SND group and in the CI group (p = 0.002558), there was no significant difference between the SND and CI groups. In the position with eyes closed (Closed), the Area parameter also significantly differed from the control both in SND and CI groups (p = 0.011060). There was no significant difference between SND and CI groups.

In children older than 8 years, there was no statistically significant difference in the values of the Area parameter between groups either in the position with eyes open (p = 0.764298) or in the position with eyes closed (p = 0.736028).

2.3 Parameter AP

In children under 8 years of age in the open-eyed position, the AP parameter was significantly higher in the CI and SND group than in the control group (p = 0.000235). In the position with eyes closed, the indices in the CI and SND groups were significantly higher than in the control group (p = 0.005888). In children older than 8 years, there were no significant differences between the groups either in the position with open eyes (p = 0.233647) or with closed eyes (p = 0.555827).

2.4 Parameter lateral

In children under 8 years of age in the position with their eyes open, the values of the Lateral parameter were significantly higher in the CI and SND group than in the control group (p = 0.001432). In the position with eyes closed, the indices in the CI group were significantly higher than in the control group (p = 0.050336). In children older than 8 years, there were no significant differences between the groups either in the position with open eyes (p = 0.255820) or with closed eyes (p = 0.920133).

2.5 Parameter AP/Lateral

Both in children under 8 years of age and over 8 years of age, there was no statistically significant difference in the values of the AP/Lateral parameter between groups neither in the position with eyes open (p = 0.993532 for the age of up to 8 years, p = 0.733826 for age over 8 years) nor in the position with eyes closed (p = 0.622120 for age up to 8 years, p = 0.764711 for age over 8 years).

2.6 Romberg Way

We did not obtain a statistically significant difference in the values of the Romberg Way parameter in children of all ages in all study groups (p = 0.157695 for the age of up to 8 years, p = 0.191010 for the age of over 8 years).

2.7 Romberg Area

We also did not obtain a statistically significant difference in the values of the Romberg Area parameter in children of all ages in all study groups (p = 0.302631 for the age of up to 8 years, p = 0.195556 for the aged over 8 years).

3. Discussion

In otology practice all over the world, there is no single consensus on the need to assess vestibular function and balance before and after cochlear implantation, and on the scope of necessary examinations. Most cochlear implant centers do not routinely assess vestibular function in the pre- and postoperative period, some - only if there are relevant complaints (dizziness, balance disorders, impaired development of motor skills), in very few - all patients undergo preoperative and postoperative vestibular testing.

Most often, the lack of vestibular testing is due to technical difficulties in examining young children and good postoperative results - children and parents rarely complain of dizziness and balance disorders.

In the literature, there are a small number of publications devoted to the assessment of postural balance in children after cochlear implantation. The results obtained are ambiguous. For example, Nair et al. when performing static posturography in children aged 2–7 years, a significant decrease in vestibular indices was revealed in the examined children after CI [21]. Kelly et al. assessed postural balance using WBB and Vestio software in 10 children aged 9–18 years after CI, revealing a significant difference in the parameters in children after CI and non-implanted children with normal hearing [22]. No significant difference was found in the parameters of postural balance in the study by Buchman et al. [23]. Walter et al. [24] found a significant improvement of postural balance parameters in bilaterally implanted patients.

Our results complement the scientific knowledge about the state of postural balance in children after cochlear implantation. In our study, children under 8 years of age after CI demonstrated a significant difference in the values of postural balance parameters in comparison with children with normal hearing. At the same time, children over eight years of age demonstrate balance indicators that do not differ significantly from those of children in the control group.

4. Conclusions

1. The Wii Balance Board with Wii Posturigrafie Software is a convenient and effective tool for assessing postural balance in children with both normal hearing and children with sensorineural deafness and after cochlear implantation.

2. In children under 8 years of age after cochlear implantation, a statistically significant increase in the values of the parameters Way, Area, AP, and Lateral in the position with open and closed eyes was revealed in comparison with children with normal hearing.

3. In children older than 8 years after cochlear implantation, there was no statistically significant difference in the values of the parameters Way, Area, AP, Lateral, AP/Lateral in the position with open and closed eyes in comparison with children with normal hearing.

4. There were no statistically significant differences in the values of the Romberg Way, and Romberg Area parameters in the children of the studied groups.

5. The study showed no difference between the parameters of postural balance in children after cochlear implantation and children with sensorineural deafness in both age groups.

Appendix

Name of parameter	Description	Units
Way	Describes the path of movement of the COP. Since the study time is set to a constant number, this parameter is characterized as the speed of COP	cm/s
Area	Marks the area and describes the variations in COP during the study	cm^2/s
Antero-Posterior (AP)	The resulting anteroposterior center of gravity vector (the length of the anteroposterior COP shifts during the study)	cm/s
Lateral	The resulting amplitude vector of the lateral displacements of the center of gravity (the length of the lateral displacements of the center of gravity during the study)	cm/s
AP/Lateral	The ratio of the anterior–posterior and lateral balance components of the subject. It reflects the general dominance of the direction of the gravitational amplitude	—

Name of parameter	Description	Units
Romberg Way	The ratio of the Way values obtained in the study with the patient's eyes open and closed	—
Romberg Area	The ratio of the Area values obtained in the study with the patient's eyes open and closed	—

Table A1.
Technical terms used in manuscript.

Author details

Maksym Situkho[1*], Viktor Lutsenko[1], Yevhen Antonov[2] and Viliam Dolinay[3]

1 Clinical Audiology and Vestibology Laboratory, Kolomiychenko Otolaryngology Institute, Kyiv, Ukraine

2 JSC Farmak, Kyiv, Ukraine

3 Faculty of Applied Informatics, Tomas Bata University, Zlín, Czechia

*Address all correspondence to: maxim.situkho@gmail.com

References

[1] Mancini M, Horak FB. The relevance of clinical balance assessment tools to differentiate balance deficits. European Journal of Physical and Rehabilitation Medicine. 2010;**46**(2):239-248

[2] Alexander NB. Postural control in older adults. Journal of the American Geriatrics Society. 1994;**42**(1):93-108

[3] Pollock AS, Durward BR, Rowe PJ, Paul JP. What is balance? Clinical Rehabilitation. 2000;**14**(4):402-406

[4] Clark RA, Bryant AL, Pua Y, McCrory P, Bennell K, et al. Validity and reliability of the Nintendo Wii Balance Board for assessment of standing balance. Gait & Posture. 2010;**31**: 307-310

[5] Park DS, Lee G. Validity and reliability of balance assessment software using the Nintendo Wii Balance Board: usability and validation. Journal of Neuroengineering and Rehabilitation. 2014;**11**:99. DOI: 10.1186/1743-0003-11-99

[6] Holmes JD, Jenkins ME, Johnson AM, Hunt MA, Clark RA. Validity of the Nintendo Wii Balance Board for the assessment of standing balance in Parkinson's disease. Clinical Rehabilitation. 2013;**27**:361-366

[7] Juneja H, Frandsen C, Nielsen NO, Larsen K, Praestegaard J. Reliability of the Wii Balance Board for measurement of steady state balance in children aged 6–9 years. Journal of Pediatric Rehabilitation Medicine. 2023;**16**(2): 1-12

[8] Jacot E, Van Den Abbeele T, Debre HR, Wiener-Vacher SR. Vestibular impairments pre- and post-cochlear implant in children. International Journal of Pediatric and Otorhinolaryngles. 2009;**73**: 209-217. DOI: 10.1016/j.ijporl.2008.10.024

[9] Zeng FG. Celebrating the one millionth cochlear implant. JASA Express Letters. 2022;**2**(7):077201

[10] O'Leary MJ, Fayad J, House WF, Linthicum FH Jr. Electrode insertion trauma in cochlear implantation. The Annals of Otology, Rhinology & Laryngology. 1991;**100**:695-699

[11] Mangham CA. Effects of cochlear prostheses on vestibuloocular reflexes to rotation. The Annals of Otology, Rhinology & Laryngology. 1987;**128**: 101-104

[12] Kubo T, Yamamoto K, Iwaki T, Doi K, Tamura M. Different forms of dizziness occurring after cochlear implant. European Archives of Otology, Rhinology & Laryngology. 2001;**258**: 9-12

[13] Tien HC, Linthicum FH Jr. Histopathologic changes in the vestibule after cochlear implantation. Otolaryngology and Head and Neck Surgery. 2002;**127**:260-264

[14] Handzel O, Burgess BJ, Nadol JB Jr. Histopathology of the peripheral vestibular system after cochlear implantation in the human. Otology & Neurotology. 2006;**27**:57-64

[15] Bance ML, O'Driscoll M, Giles E, Ramdsen RT. Vestibular stimulation by multichannel cochlear implants. Laryngoscope. 1998;**108**: 291-294

[16] Wu Q, Zhang Q, Xiao Q, Zhang Y, Chen Z, Liu S, et al. Vestibular

dysfunction in pediatric patients with cochlear implantation: A systematic review and meta-analysis. Frontiers in Neurology. 2022;**13**:996580

[17] Pivnickova L, Vasek V, Dolinay V, editors. Numerical Methods of the Examination of the Postural Stability. Vienna: DAAAM International; 2011

[18] Pivnickova L, Dolinay V, Vasek V. The Wii balance board as a tool for evaluation of the static computed posturography. International Journal of Circuits, Systems and Signal Processing. 2014;**8**:607-615

[19] Shumway-Cook A, Woollacott MH. The growth of stability: postural control from a development perspective. Journal of Motor Behavior. 1985;**17**(2):131-147

[20] Bourelle S, Dey N, Sifaki-Pistolla D, Berge B, Gautheron V, Cottalorda J, et al. Computerized static posturography and laterality in children: Influence of age. Acta Bioengineering and Biomechanical. 2017;**19**(2):129-139

[21] Nair S, Gupta A, Nilakantan A, Mittal R, Dahiya R, Saini S, et al. Impaired vestibular function after cochlear implantation in children: Role of static posturography. Indian Journal of Otolaryngology and Head Neck Surgery. 2017;**69**(2):252-258

[22] Kelly A, Liu Z, Leonard S, Toner F, Adams M, Toner J. Balance in children following cochlear implantation. Cochlear Implants International. 2018; **19**(1):22-25. DOI: 10.1080/14670100.2017.1379180

[23] Buchman CA, Joy J, Hodges A, Telischi FF, Balkany TJ. Vestibular effects of cochlear implantation. Laryngoscope. 2004;**114**(10):1-22. DOI: 10.1097/00005537-200,410, 001-00001

[24] Wolter Nikolaus E, Gordon Karen A, Campos Jennifer L, et al. Head-referenced cochlear implant stimulation improves balance in children with bilateral cochleovestibular loss. Audiology and Neurotology. 2019; **25**(1–2):60-71

Chapter 9

Auditory Neuropathy Spectrum Disorder: Genetic and Electrophysiological Testing for Predicting Rehabilitation Outcomes after Cochlear Implantation

Maria Lalayants

Abstract

Reviling the etiology or at least pathophysiology of auditory neuropathy spectrum disorder is crucial for choosing rehabilitation pathway and predicting rehabilitation outcomes. Some patients with auditory neuropathy spectrum disorder undergo cochlear implantation, but it is not always possible to foresee the results of rehabilitation. Genetic testing, especially in cases without obviously perinatal hearing loss risk factors, might help to understand etiology and pathophysiology, whether it is synaptopathy or neuropathy; therefore, it becomes possible to predict rehabilitation outcomes. More than 20 genes related to auditory neuropathy spectrum disorder phenotype are known already. Modern genetic approaches, such as whole genome and whole exome sequencing, reveal etiology of auditory neuropathy spectrum disorder in many cases. But there are still auditory neuropathy spectrum disorder cases with unknown etiology and site of the lesion. Electrophysiological methods (electrocochleography, electrically evoked brainstem potentials) might help to localize the site of lesion in hearing system and therefore help to predict rehabilitation outcomes. Electrically evoked brainstem potential testing after cochlear implantation seems to be applicable and useable tool to predict potential CI outcomes and to choose optimal rehabilitation trace.

Keywords: auditory neuropathy spectrum disorder, cochlear implantation, auditory synaptopathy, Otoferlin, genetic testing, electrically evoked brainstem potentials, eABR, ANSD

1. Introduction

Auditory neuropathy spectrum disorder (ANSD) is an electrophysiological label, that incorporates patients with hearing loss of different etiologies and pathogenesis but united based on the presence of pre-neural cochlear responses such as otoacoustic emission (OAE) and cochlear microphonics (CM) and absent or grossly abnormal auditory brain steam responses (ABRs). This electrophysiological picture might reflect the presence of pathology of the auditory system of various etiologies in any site in the auditory system from the inter hair cells (IHC) to the brain stem (including synapses, dendrites of spiral ganglion neurons, spiral ganglion neurons themselves, the auditory nerve). Therefore, ANSD is characterized by a different course and results of rehabilitation, which in many cases are difficult to predict. Elucidating the etiology and/or patophysiology of hearing loss mechanisms in these children might help to choose an optimal rehabilitation approach and predict rehabilitation outcomes [1, 2].

2. Etiology of auditory neuropathy spectrum disorder

Despite of electrophysiological commonality of ANSD, there is a broad spectrum of audiological clinical features, which come from different possible pathophysiological mechanisms due to different etiology of ANSD. About half of the cases of ANSD in children are diagnosed in those who were born premature. ANSD risk is higher among children that were born at 32 or earlier gestational week. The mechanism of ANSD among these children is due to incomplete myelinization and affected inner hair cells, as it was demonstrated in postmortem histology -inner hair cells were affected much more than outer hair cells. Also, risk factors for the development of ANSD include hyperbilirubinemia, congenital cytomegalovirus infection, asphyxia, and low birth weight. Genetic testing of patients with ANSD during the last two and half decades revealed more than 20 genes associated with that type of hearing loss. MRI testing reviled that the electrophysiological picture of congenital ANSD might be also due to the hypoplastic cochlear nerve (cochlear nerve deficiency). ANSD might be also acquired letter in life as a result of late-onset genetic-based mechanisms or due to an autoimmune reaction [3–6].

Despite of progress and availability of modern genetic tests and imaging technologies, the etiology of many cases of congenital or acquired ANSD is still unknown.

3. Broad clinical and audiological phenotype of auditory neuropathy spectrum disorder

In addition to the two main electrophysiological features mentioned above, the clinical and audiological picture of ANSD is characterized by:

1. Thresholds of pure tone audiometry can vary from normal to profound, fluctuate, and do not correspond to ABR data.

2. Violation, first of all, of speech recognition, especially in difficult acoustic situations, tone-speech dissociation (dissociation of the degree of speech recognition impairment with the thresholds of pure tone audiometry).

3. Auditory steady-state response (ASSR) are recordable in patients with ANSD, but they do not meet both the ABR thresholds (mostly absent) and the thresholds of pure tone audiometry.

Thus, objective methods of audiological examination make it possible to establish the diagnosis of ANSD, but they do not allow to establish either the degree of hearing loss or the shape of the audiogram. As long as, in patients with ANSD, behavioral thresholds for the perception of sounds can correspond to varying degrees of hearing loss from mild or even close to normal to profound, some patients with ANSD do not require even hearing aids, while others might require cochlear implants. At the same time, it is necessary to take into account that patients with ANSD with profound impairment of speech recognition, which does not correspond to the degree of hearing loss might become a candidate for cochlear implantation despite the degree of hearing loss. Choosing the optimal rehabilitation method is also complicated by the fluctuation of hearing thresholds in some patients, as well as the possibility of hearing improvement in others, primarily those prematurely born, with ANSD during the first 1–2 years of age. Nevertheless, many patients with ANSD undergo cochlear implantation, but it is not always possible to foresee the results of rehabilitation without understanding the pathophysiological mechanism of hearing deficit [7–9].

Pathophysiological mechanisms of ANSD according to localization of pathology in auditory pathway might be divided into two groups – auditory synaptopathy and auditory neuropathy (**Figure 1**). In the case of auditory synaptopathy, pathology is localized in inner hair cells, synapses between inner hair cells and spiral ganglion neurons (SNG) dendrites, or in dendrites itself. In these cases, we might predispose that SNG cells and cochlear nerve are preserved and electrical stimulation of the spiral ganglion through cochlear implant will compensate hearing deficit. While in the case of auditory neuropathy type of ANSD, which is due to myelinopathy or axonopathy, or hypoplastic cochlear nerve, the site of lesion is located more proximal than site of electrical stimulation through CI, therefore hearing impairment is difficult to be compensated by cochlear implant electrical stimulation [10–13].

Lack of data on the mechanism of development of ANSD in each case, with a variety of clinical and audiological manifestations of ANSD in general, is the main reason for the difficulties in classifying ANSD. At the moment there is no universally accepted, optimal classification of ANSD.

Several variants of the ANSD classification have been proposed: according to the clinical picture; localization of the pathology etcetera. For example, presynaptic and

Synaptophaty	presynaptic (OTOF, SLC17A8, CACNA1D, CABP2 genes) postsynaptic (OPA1, DIAPH3, ATP1A3 genes)
Neuropathy	Charcot-Marie-Tooth Syndrome (MPZ, PMP22, NDRG1, NFEL, GJB1, GJB3 genes), Friedreich'sAtaxia (FXN gene), Wolfram syndrome (WFS1 gene), Mohr Tranebjerg Syndrome (TIMM8A gene), COWCK Syndrome (AIFM1 gene) , Leigh syndrome (NARS2 gene)

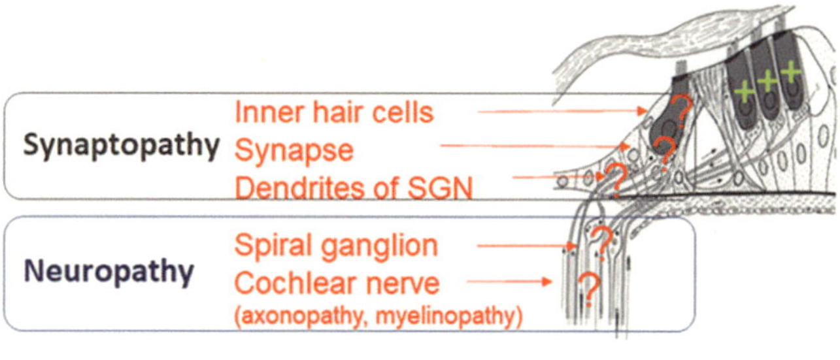

Figure 1.
Auditory synaptopathy and auditory neuropathy: Genetic cause and site of lesion.

postsynaptic. It was also proposed to highlight more detailed options: synaptopathy, ganglionopathy, myelinopathy, and axonopathy. However, classification according to such detailed morphological features, while the histological examination is impossible, can mainly be done only when a genetic mechanism is identified.

Subdivision of ANSD into synaptopathies and neuropathies seems to be the most practical. Firstly, such classification makes it possible to predict the results of cochlear implantation, and secondly, genetically determined auditory synaptopathies usually lead to the development of an isolated (nonsyndromic) hearing impairment, while genetic disorders leading to the development of neuropathy type of ANSD are most often accompanied by damage to other nerves, which might lead to syndromic form of hearing loss.

When cochlear nerve deficiency is excluded by MRI, there are two main approaches two distinguish auditory synaptopathy and neuropathy: genetic testing and electrophysiological testing.

4. Genetic cause of ANSD

More than 20 genes related to ANSD phenotype are known already. Some of them cause isolated ANSD, others—syndromic ANSD. Inheritance of ANSD can be dominant, recessive, X-linked, or mitochondrial. According to the site of lesion—genetically related auditory synaptopathy or—genetically related auditory neuropathy. Synaptophaty cases might be also divided into presynaptic or postsynaptic synaptopathy.

Genetically related ANSD can be isolated or syndromic. Mutation in SLC17A8 and DIAPH3 might cause isolated ANSD, but most cases of isolated ANSD are related to the OTOF gene mutations. Syndromic ANSD is associated with peripheral neuropathy, optic atrophy and has been linked with mutations in genes leading to Friedreich's Ataxia, Charcot-Marie-Tooth Syndrome, Leber's Optic Atrophy, Mohr Tranebjerg Syndrome, and others.

The synaptopathy type of ANSD is quite often nonsyndromic due to the unique structure of the synapses between the internal hair cells (IHCs) and the peripheral processes of the spiral ganglion neurons. They differ from synapses in the central nerve system, primarily because of synaptic bodies (ribbon synapses), resembling similar structures in retinal synapses, but which are characterized by the presence of molecules unique specifically for the auditory system. Synaptic ribbon at the presynaptic membrane holds many presynaptic vesicles with a neurotransmitter. With sound stimulation, displacement of the stereocilia of the IHCs—mechanosensitive cation channels open—cations, primarily K ions, enter the IHC, which leads to depolarization of the IHC and the opening of voltage-dependent calcium channels. Molecules of Otoferlin, located near synaptic bodies, when interacting with calcium ions, maintain the rapid simultaneous exocytosis of many presynaptic vesicles with glutamate, which ensure the transmission of the temporal aspects of an acoustic stimulus. In addition to the mentioned Otoferlin, there are other unique components in the synaptic transmission in the IHC. For example, pinocytosis (reabsorption of glutamate from the synaptic cleft) in the IHC is provided by VGluT3, unlike synapses in other structures using VGluT1 or VGluT2. The calcium channel complex also contains structures that are unique only for IHC —Ca1.3 L. The uniqueness of VGluT3, Otoferlin, and other, but not all, components of synaptic transmission in the IHC, in case of corresponding gene mutation, underline isolated form of ANSD—other organs and systems are not affected.

The proximal portion of the terminal dendrites of SGN, as well as axons in the area closer to the SG, are wrapped in Schwann cells. At the entrance to the brainstem, the axons of SGN are wrapped in oligodendrocytes. Genetic impairments in the functional consistency of these structures, primarily Schwann cells, can make it difficult to conduct a nerve impulse through SGN, especially temporal characteristics of a sound stimulus, which is primarily manifested by impaired speech recognition. Schwann cells and oligodendrocytes are also found in other parts of the nervous system, therefore in these cases, auditory neuropathy is usually not isolated, it is combined with lesions in other organs and systems. Impaired myelination, for example, in various types of Charcot-Marie-Tooth syndrome, is accompanied by a slowdown in conduction along the auditory nerve, which can, in particular, lead to impaired localization of sounds, and speech recognition, especially in noise.

So, in the case of auditory synaptopathy, the uniqueness of the corresponding synapses explains the non-syndromic nature of ANSD in most cases. Localization of the site of the lesion in the cochlear organ of Corti allows to predict satisfactory results of rehabilitation by cochlear implantation (with intact SG and overlying structures). In auditory neuropathy involving SGN, myelination may be impaired due to the pathology of Schwann cells, common in the human nervous system, which, in most cases, is accompanied by the involvement of other structures of the nervous system. Violation of the myelination of the auditory nerve, dyssynchronization is often manifested by a violation of speech recognition. Localization of the pathology is such cases does not allow one to expect satisfactory results of rehabilitation after cochlear implantation.

Genetic testing especially in cases without obvious perinatal hearing loss risk factors might help to understand etiology, pathophysiology, whether it is synaptopathy or neuropathy, and therefore, it becomes possible to predict rehabilitation outcomes.

This list of ANSD-related genes in **Figure 1** is not complete yet. A modern genetic approach, such as whole genome and whole exome sequencing, reveals new gene candidates for ANSD.

4.1 Auditory synaptopathies

Genes that lead to the development of synaptopathies, can be divided to two subgroups: presynaptic synaptopathy genes (impairment at the level of IHC, glutamate exocytosis) and postsynaptic synaptopathy genes (impairment of excitation of the dendrites of SGN). The genes for presynaptic synaptopathy include OTOF, SLC17A8, CACNA1D, and CABP2. Accordingly, these patients are promising candidates for rehabilitation by cochlear implantation. Postsynaptic synaptopathy genes include OPA1, DIAPH3, and ATP1A3. Despite that, these genes cause impairment at the level of dendrites of SGN, the body and axons of SGN and their myelinization seem to be preserved and electrical stimulation through cochlear implant might lead to good outcomes of rehabilitation.

4.1.1 OTOF gene, Otoferlin protein

According to the literature, the most common hereditary cause of ANSD is mutations in the OTOF gene encoding the Otoferlin protein. The OTOF gene and Otoferlin protein were first described in 1999. Otoferlin is expressed in the inner ear and the brain of humans. This is a calcium-dependent protein, the main function of which is the exocytosis of presynaptic vesicles with the neurotransmitter glutamate into the synaptic cleft. More than 100 mutations have already been described in the OTOF gene, 75% of which are inactivating, leading to the absence of Otoferlin and therefore impaired synaptic transmission in the inner ear. Patients with biallelic inactivating mutations in the OTOF gene are diagnosed with bilateral non-syndromic autosomal recessive severe hearing loss (DFNB9) with an electrophysiological pattern of ANSD. The rest of the mutations are non-inactivating and lead to the synthesis of a functionally defective protein. In most cases, they lead to congenital severe hearing loss, however, cases of mild HL and even temperature-sensitive HL have been described in patients with some inactivating OTOF gene mutations—hearing thresholds are within or close to normal range, but there may be some impairment of speech recognition, especially in noise. With an increase in body temperature, sometimes even by 1°C, the patient's hearing deteriorates, while when the temperature normalizes, the hearing threshold is restored. Mutations in the OTOF gene are responsible for the development of 1.4–5% of cases of congenital non-syndromic sensorineural hearing loss, according to studies in various countries [14–16].

In different countries, there is genetic heterogeneity in the prevalence of mutations in general and the mutation profile of the OTOF gene, in particular. Thus, in Spain, the Glu829Ter mutation of the OTOF gene is not only a common cause of ANSD but is also the third most common cause of non-syndromic prelingual SNHL in general—it was detected in almost 8% of cases. In a study of the contribution of OTOF mutations to the incidence of SNHL in Japan biallelic mutations in the OTOF gene were found in 1.7% of cases, while not a single patient with the Glu829Ter mutation was found. OTOF variants, including a founder variant (p.Arg1939Gln) among Koreans, account for approximately 90% of Korean prelingual ANSD cases with anatomically intact cochlear nerves. In Russia, genetic testing of 50 children with ANSD without cochlear nerve aplasia revealed biallelic mutation of the OTOF in 12 children (24% of cases). Otoacoustic emission was recordable in all children until the last examination at the age of 12 years. In one case OAE was partly preserved even in the implanted ear 10 years after CI. No improvement, or fluctuations in hearing thresholds were noted. Ten children with OTOF-related ANSD underwent cochlear implantation, including a child with mild hearing loss, but dramatically impaired speech recognition. After cochlear implantation, the action potential of the auditory nerve to electrical stimulation and electrically evoked brainstem responses were recordable in all tested cases due to preserved cochlear nerve and the auditory pathway of the brain steam. Rehabilitation outcomes in these patients are comparable to other patients with cochlear hearing loss, like GJB2-related HL. These data are consistent with other literature describing good outcomes of CI in patients with OTOF-related ANSD [7, 13, 17, 18].

The prevalence of OTOF-related ANSD and good outcomes of CI make the search for mutations in the OTOF gene the essential component of the genetic examination of patients with ANSD, especially in early childhood hearing loss. Testing for the OTOF gene is included in many protocols for the management of children with ANSD, and the OTOF gene is included in most existing MPS gene panels for hearing loss.

The other genes that are associated with presynaptic synaptopathy, were described just in several cases now.

4.1.2 SLC17A8 gene, VGLUT3 protein: Vesicular glutamate transporter 3

Mutations in the SLC17A8 gene lead to postlingual progressive, predominantly high frequency, autosomal dominant nonsyndromic HL in humans. A study on mice showed that in mice knocked out by the slc17a8 gene synaptic transmission is impaired due to a lack of glutamate exocytosis. At the same time, eABR were recordable, which reflected intact SGN and overlying structures and the prospects for CI as a method of rehabilitation [19].

4.1.3 CACNA1D, calcium voltage-gated channel subunit alpha1D (Cav1.3) protein

The CACNA1D gene encodes the α1 subunit involved in the formation of calcium channel pores Ca1.3. The gene is expressed in hair cells, cardiomyocytes, neurons, and neuroendocrine cells, therefore mutations in the CACNA1D gene develop a syndromic form of ANSD - prelingual hearing loss with sinoatrial node dysfunction (SANND) [20, 21].

4.1.4 CABP2, calcium-binding protein 2

CABP2, Calcium-binding protein 2, is involved in calcium entry through Ca1.3 channels. Hearing impairment in patients with a mutation in the CABP2 gene is prelingual, and moderately severe, combined with Marfan-like features in the patient [22].

4.1.5 OPA1 gene, mitochondrial dynamin-related GTPase protein

According to the literature, the most common hereditary cause of postsynaptic synaptopathy type of ANSD is mutations in OPA1 gene, which encodes the Mitochondrial dynamin-related GTPase protein. This protein is located in the inner membrane of mitochondria and is involved in many processes in the cell. Mutations in the OPA1 gene can lead to the development of non-syndromic dominant optic atrophy without hearing loss (DOA) or to dominant optic atrophy with hearing loss (DOA+). Most of the known mutations causing haploinsufficiency lead to the development of non-syndromic DOA. While, missense mutations, primarily Arg445His, probably through a dominant negative effect, lead to the formation of dominant optic atrophy with hearing loss (DOA+) Hearing impairment, in this case, is usually postlingval, after the manifestation of visual impairment. Hearing loss is progressive, of varying degrees, and audiogram profile, even within the same family. Electrocochleography in patients with DOA+, as well as studies in mice, suggested that the OHC and IHC were preserved, but the dendrites of SGN were damaged. Electrically evoked cochlear nerve action potential and eABR after cochlear implantation are recordable in patients with OPA1-related ANSD, which proved that SGN and cochlear nerve were intact in these patients. The results of cochlear implantation in patients with DOA+ are satisfactory [23, 24].

4.1.6 DIAPH3, Diaphanousformin 3 protein

The function of Diaphanusformin 3, encoded by the DIAPH3 gene, is not completely clear. However, overexpression of this gene leads to damage to SGN dendrites. A study on mice also showed the possibility of involvement in the pathological process of IHC stereocilia. Hearing impairment was postlingual, and progressive, with an autosomal dominant mode of inheritance. Satisfactory results of CI have been described in several implanted patients [25].

4.1.7 ATP1A3, Alpha-3 protein

ATP1A3 encodes Alpha-3 protein catalytic subunit of the Na+/K + ATP transmembrane ion pump that provides the resting membrane potential. The ATP1A3 gene is expressed in the peripheral processes of SGN, in the basal ganglia, the hypocampus, and the cerebellum, therefore mutations in the ATP1A3 gene can lead to the development of the syndromic ANSD—CAPOS syndrome (hearing loss, cerebellar ataxia, areflexia, optic atrophy, cavus pes). Cases with non-syndromic HL were also described.CI in patients with mutations in the ATP1A3 gene, due to the localization of the lesion at the level of peripheral processes of SGN, led to good outcomes of rehabilitation [26].

4.2 Auditory neuropathies

Mutations in genes leading to the development of polyneuropathies cause "true" auditory neuropathies with damage to spiral ganglion neurons and/or demyelination of auditory nerve fibers. Auditory neuropathy-type hearing loss has been described in some patients with mutations in mitochondrial genes: MTND4 (Leber's syndrome), TMEM126A. The largest group of patients with auditory neuropathy type of ANSD is Charcot-Marie-Tooth syndrome [10, 11, 13, 27, 28].

Charcot-Marie-Tooth syndrome (CMT), or hereditary motor sensory neuropathies, is a clinically and genetically heterogeneous group of slowly progressive hereditary neuropathies with wide phenotype variation. CMT syndrome can be inherited in an autosomal dominant, autosomal recessive, or X-linked manner. Mutations in more than 60 genes can cause CMT, but mutations in the PMP22, MPZ, GJB1, and MFN2 genes are the most common.

The clinical picture is dominated by distal muscle wasting and weakness, decreased tendon reflexes, and distal, usually symmetrical, desensitization. Patients with CMT may also have signs of damage to other nerves, leading, respectively, the visual impairments in the form of optical atrophy, atrophy of the tongue, dysfunction of the vocal cords, diaphragm, as well as hearing loss. Sensorineural hearing loss has been described in cases related to mutations in these genes: MPZ, PMP22, NEFL, SH3TC2, NDRG1, GJB1, AIFM1, PRPS1 and INF2. Considering the pathophysiology of disorders in CMT syndrome, myelinopathy and axonopathy, it can be assumed that in patients with CMT, hearing loss will be in form of auditory neuropathy. However, in most cases, the examination of patients with CMT is limited with PTA and does not include the recording of ABR, therefore, auditory neuropathy in these cases might be missed. Moreover, even in cases where the data of pure-tone audiometry are within the normal range, auditory neuropathy cannot be excluded in a patient without registration of ABR, especially since some patients have impaired speech recognition, especially in noise. Among above-listed genes associated with hearing loss in CMT the most frequent is the MPZ gene [28–30].

4.2.1 MPZ gene, Myelin protein-zero

MPZ gene encodes Myelin protein-zero and is expressed only in Schwann cells. The main type of mutation is the point. In a patient with a mutation in the MPZ gene and HL, a considerable lesion of ganglion cells and auditory nerve fibers with a preserved IHC and practically intact OHC were described. The MPZ protein plays an important but complex role in myelination. One of the functions of MPZ, which has been confirmed by many studies, is the mediation of the process of myelin compaction through the adhesion of opposing membrane structures. MPZ acts as a homophilic molecule, the extracellular portion of which, expressed on one membrane surface, can interact with a similar region of the same protein expressed on another membrane surface. Mice in which MPZ expression was inactivated had non-compacted myelin sheaths and severe peripheral neuropathy. Therefore, mutations in regions of the MPZ responsible for protein-protein interaction cause a more severe clinical phenotype than mutations in other regions. MPZ also has a regulatory function in the myelination process. Mice in which MPZ expression has been inactivated have dysregulated myelin gene expression and malposition of several non-compacted myelin proteins.

Hearing impairment as well as pupillary abnormalities have been described in Asp75Val and Thr124Met mutations - CMT type 2 J. With Glu97Val mutation in patients with CMT 2 J. Seeman et al. (2004) noted that hearing loss may appear up to 10 years before the onset of muscle weakness. Mild hearing loss has been noted with the Pro105Thr mutation. The disease usually manifests in the 2nd or 3rd decade of life and has a progressive course. Since, in most cases, registration of ABRs was not used to examine patients, the diagnosis of auditory neuropathy could not be detected [31].

A comprehensive survey of families with the Tyr145Ser mutation in MPZ was performed by Starr A. et al. (2003). The audiological examination included registration of ABR, OAE, cortical potentials, and psychoacoustic tests, which made it possible to describe auditory neuropathy in family members with the mutation. Pathological and histological examinations revealed not only demyelination but also a decrease in the number of spiral ganglion neurons by more than 90%. At the same time, OHC and IHC were preserved (but in the apex of the cochlea, the number of OHC was reduced). In the described cases of cochlear implantation, despite the improvement in sound perception, CI does not lead to a significant improvement in speech perception, probably due to the death of SG neurons described by Arnold Starr [30].

4.2.2 PMP22

PMP22 gene encodes a 22-kD protein that comprises from 2 to 5% of peripheral nervous system myelin. It is produced primarily by Schwann cells and expressed in the compact portion of essentially all myelinated fibers in the peripheral nervous system. The main type of mutations in PMP22 are duplications (up to 3–4 copies) as a result of unequal crossing over.

Mild to moderate sensorineural hearing loss, with greater loss in the low and high frequencies, has been described in patients with various types of mutations in the PMP22 gene. In patients with a duplication, hearing loss is congenital and less prone to a progressive course. Hearing loss in patients with a deletion of the PMP22 site, leading to hereditary neuropathy with a tendency to pressure palsies, occurred in the second decade of life and a tendency to a progressive course. However, speech recognition was not as impaired as with mutations in the MPZ gene. Thus, according to Verhagen W (2005), speech audiometry in examined patients with mutations in the PMP22 gene corresponded to tone threshold audiometry [32].

CI in a patient with PMP22-related ANSD demonstrated improvements in speech discrimination scores, however, they do not achieve the results in the typical subset of patients receiving CI [33].

In patients with CMT, cochlear implantation may reconstitute synchronous neural activity by way of supraphysiological electrical stimulation, so they can get some benefit from CI, although not at the same level as patients with cochlear hearing loss.

4.2.3 Other syndromes with ANSD

ANSD type of hearing loss can be diagnosed in patients with Friedreich's syndrome (FXN gene) - mild hearing loss, mainly impaired speech intelligibility. In such patients, the effectiveness of the use of FM systems was noted [34].

Some mutations in the WFS1 gene can lead to the development of Wolfram's syndrome, with early childhood and congenital hearing loss, predominantly low-frequency, with diabetes and visual impairment, with an autosomal recessive type of inheritance. Other mutations lead to low-frequency hearing loss, which is inherited in an autosomal dominant manner [35].

Mutations in the TIMM8A gene lead to the development of Mohr-Tranimerg syndrome with prelingual hearing loss. Optic neuropathy, atony and paranoia appear in the second decade of life, with progressive neurodegeneration [36].

Mutations in the AIFM1 gene lead to COWCK syndrome - prellingual hearing loss, progressive neuromuscular and cognitive impairments, and progressive hypoplasia of the auditory nerve [37].

Leigh's syndrome with a progressive neurodegenerative lesion of the central nervous system and hearing loss develops due to mutations in the NARS2 gene [38].

Auditory neuropathy type ANSD and progressive neurodegenerotion do not allow to expect satisfactory results of cochlear implantation in patients with these syndromes.

Auditory neuropathy-type hearing loss has been described in some patients with mutations in mitochondrial genes: MTND4 (Leber's syndrome), TMEM126A [39].

Modern massively parallel sequencing based methods allows to find more and more new ANSD causative genes, which previously were not associated with ANSD. For example, recently two mutations were found in TWNK gene of our 8-year-old patient with ANSD.

Mutations in TWNK gene were described in patients with Perrault syndrome - autosome-recessive disease, which includes sensorineural hearing loss, cerebellar ataxia, motor and sensory neuropathy, ovarian dysfunction, opftalmoplegiya. But previously HL was not described as ANSD in TWNK related disorders. After CI the EABRS were not recordable in our patients, speech recognition was poor. These data and patophisiology of TWNK related disorders, which is based on axonopathy, lead to conclusion, that TWNK-related ANSD cause auditory neuropathy type of ANSD [40].

Patients with auditory neuropathy type of ANSD due to mutations described above might get some benefit from CI, but in most cases they do not achieve the level of rehabilitation outcomes of patients with auditory synaptopathy and cochlear HL. The possibility of a poor outcomes of CI should be discussed with patient and patients caregiver before CI.

5. Methods of genetic testing

First of all, genetic testing is highly indicated for patients with a family history of hearing loss. The probability of identifying the genetic nature of ANSD is significantly higher in the group of patients without perinatal risk factors for hearing loss and cochlear nerve deficiency on MRI.

Despite of prevalence of OTOF gene mutation among patients with ANSD, it does not as high as GJB2 gene mutation prevalence in congenital "cochlear" SNHL. Therefore, single gene testing is not rationale in case of ANSD.

Development of massively parallel sequencing (MPS) and creation of multigene panels, including panels on hearing loss, containing several dozens of "hearing loss genes", as well as the development and availability of the whole genome and whole exome sequencing method, is a promising direction in the genetic examination of patients with auditory neuropathy spectrum disease, which makes it possible to identify rare forms of hereditary hearing loss.

There are 4 main types of MPS based methods (**Figure 2**):

MPS panels (NGS gene panel).

Clinical exome sequencing.

Whole exome sequencing (WES).

Whole genome sequencing (WGS).

The complete genomic information within a sample or individual is known as the whole genome. Exons are the genome's protein-coding regions and are collectively known as the exome. Despite the exome's relatively small proportion of the whole genome (approximately 2%), exomes encode most known disease-related variants. Clinical Exome Sequencing is a test for identifying disease-causing DNA variants within the 1% of the genome which codes for proteins (exons) or flanks the regions which code for proteins (splice junctions). MPS gene panels are more targeted and analyze only known disease-associated genes for specific diseases. The advantages of panels over WES or WGS include lower cost, simpler analysis, and optimisation of variant detection in the included genes. Disadvantages include the inability to analyze or re-analyze genes not included on the MPS panel. Nevertheless, gene panels that include at least OTOF gene might be the first line genetic testing of patients with ANSD. Whereas WES or even better WGS may be second-line testing options.

WGS or at least WES are better options than clinical exome sequencing, because of genetic heterogeneity of ANSD and there are still a lot of genes and mutations to be reviled as a cause of ANSD.

The main advantages of Whole Genome Sequencing

- Analyze the whole genome, including coding, non-coding, and mitochondrial DNA
- Discover novel genomic variants (structural, single nucleotide, insertion-deletion, copy number)
- Identify previously unknown variants for future targeted studies
- Possibility re-analyze data when there is new information on the genetic cause of disease

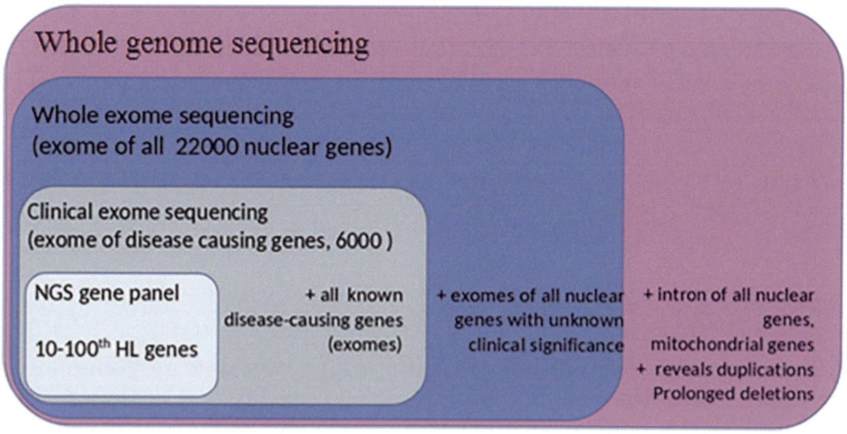

Figure 2.
Massively parallel sequencing based methods and their relationship.

The main disadvantage of WES and especially WGS is their cost and the complexity of data interpretation. Nevertheless, these methods serve an as important tool for reviling ANSD etiology in tested children and for data collection for a better understanding of ANSD mechanism in patients to come.

5.1 What if genetic testing does not revile the etiology and patophysiology of ANSD?

Even all above-described methods do not give clues in many cases. Some electrophysiological methods might help to localize the site of lesion in hearing system and therefore help to predict rehabilitation outcomes. First of all, it is electrocochleography. Presence, absence, or changes in different components of electrocochleography reflects the pathology in cochlea. Electrically evoked brainstem potentials (eABR) reflect the integrity of the hearing system up to brain steam when nerve impulse in cochlear nerve is derived by electrical stimulation. These data help to predict CI outcomes even if the etiology of hearing loss is unknown. When brainstem response to electrical stimuli is present—good CI outcomes might be expected. While eABR absence does not allow to expect good rehabilitation outcomes. Both of these methods require a stimulation electrode to be placed on the promontorium of the cochlea to achieve the clearest and reliable data. In the case of small children, these invasive procedures require sedation. If the test results indicate on electable eABR (probably synaptopathy type of ANSD), that would encourage audiologists and parents to provide cochlear implantation. But even if the test result is negative—it does not exclude cochlear implantation as an option for that child and the patient still might benefit from CI. Therefore these invasive, requiring sedation methods are not fully justified. On the other hand, EABR testing after cochlear implantation seems to be useable tool to predict CI outcomes and chose optimal rehabilitation trace after CI [41].

6. Electrically evoked auditory brainsteam responses

Electrically evoked auditory brainstem responses are bioelectrical responses from auditory pathway up to the level of the brainstem to electrical stimuli. Stimulating electrode might be situated at the promontorium, in round window night, but the largest response can be achieved when the electrode is located as close as possible to the spiral ganglion and auditory nerve. Therefore, intracochlear electrodes of CI are the best. EABR testing after CI reflects retrocochlear development after initiation of CI-mediated electrical stimulation, integrity of neural response to CI stimulation, and functional status of auditory pathway up to the brainstem. EABRs after CI can be used for verifying devise and electrode function and can assist in sound processors fitting to some extent [42, 43].

6.1 EABRs testing and morphology

EABRs might be recorded using specific for certain CI system programming software and hardware to provide stimuli (Custom SoundEP for Cochlear, SCLIN for Advanced Bionics, Maestro for Med-El) and a clinical system for evoked potentials registration. These two systems should be connected by trigger cable to synchronize stimulation and ABRs registration (**Figure 3**).

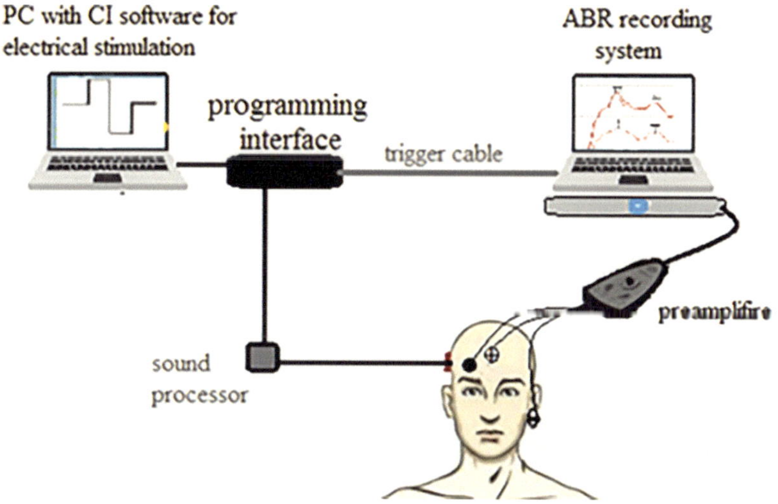

Figure 3.
EABRs recording setup.

Stimulus that is used to elict the eABRs is usually a single biphasic current pulse delivered at a repetition rate as in acoustically evoked ABR. For stimulation bipolar or monopolar electrode coupling mode might be used. Monopolar – active electrode is one of the intracochlear electrodes and indeferent electrode is extracochlear. This mode allows getting more electrode and tonotopically-specific responses. While bipolar stimulation with both intracochlear active and indeferent electrode lead to a "click"-like stimulation, which helps to elict larger response [42–45].

EABRs just as acoustically evoked ABR consist of waves II-V and usually are marked as eII-eV. Waves VI-VII usually are not seen. Wave I and sometimes wave II are consiled by stimulus artifact. There are some specific parameters and morphology of EABRs:

EABR wave latencies are 1–2 ms earlier than in ABR (but interpeak intervals are the same).

Wave V latency is approximately 4.0 ms and does not change much with an intensity of stimulation (about 0,4 ms shift between upper comfort and threshold level).

Wave V latency tends to be shorter for apical electrodes, than for basal electrodes [45].

Different parameters of eABRs were measured to asses neural response properties. First of all, eABRS thresholds. They are higher than the minimum level of electric stimulation that evokes sound sensation. This difference comes from a difference in the rate of stimulation: 25–50 stimulus per second for eABRs and 900–3000 per second for speech processor stimulation map. Therefore, eABRs, unlike ABRs, cannot be used for setting stimulation threshold levels during sound processor fitting.

Other parameters might be also explored: peak and interpeak latencies, amplitude growth function (obtained by the response amplitude, usually eV, as a function of stimulation level); channel interaction (by simultaneous stimulation of two electrode pairs); electrode positioning (lower eABR thresholds for an electrode placed near to modiolus). Waves eV and eIII latencies degrees during the first year after CI, which reflects auditory nerve and brainstem development after CI. Interestingly, there was no effect of age of CI on latency change. But despite all those parameters, the main prognostic value has eABRs present itself. The presence of eABRs is a good prognostic sign for CI outcomes, at least it might be concluded that peripheral hearing deficiency might be compensated. This is especially important in cases of CI-challenging patients such as patients with cochlear malformation and, of course, with ANSD [45–47].

6.2 EABR testing in patients with ANSD

Several research groups during the last twenty years have studied eABR features in patients with ANSD. Some studies had showed reduced suprathreshold eV and neural dyssynchrony in patients with ANSD. The most interesting area of these research was the relationship between eABRs and speech perception after CI.

Researches compared eABRs after CI in patients with ANSD and without. It was shown that the eABR threshold and suprathreshold amplitude measures were more variable in patients with ANSD. Nevertheless, eABRs were measurable in most cases and proved that CI can provide synchronous neural responses to auditory stimulation in ANSD. EABR measures indicated that subjects with ANSD have sufficient neural sensitivity to electrical stimulation, however, they may experience less robust neural responses at suprathreshold levels. Variability in eABR parameters was most probably related to different etiology and patophysiology of ANSD.

The outcome of cochlear implantation in those patients with ANSD with recordable eABRs were not significantly different from that in other pediatric implant patients. But patients with absent eABR or with just even abnormal eABRs wave morphology had significantly worse speech outcomes. Physiologic data suggest that generally, the CI can overcome the desynchronization or whatsoever underlying ANSD and eABRs waveform are a predictor of postoperative outcomes [45–49].

EABRs were investigated in patients with ANSD with known etiology, mostly in genetically related cases.

Hosoya M. 2018 observed elongated eV wave in patients with OTOF-related ANSD. But this eV latency elongation did not affect negatively speech perception and CI outcomes. The same observation we had testing our 8 patients with OTOF-related ANSD - EABRs were recordable right after the sound processor first fitting, but even 10 years later eV latency in OTOF-related child is larger than in his pears with for example prematurity related ANSD. These data indicate that Otoferlin might play role in neurotransmission in more central part of auditory pathway than just in IHC synapses. Although there is no evidence of OTOF expression in central neural system in humans, OTOF expression was reported in rats' cerebellum [50].

EABR registration in OPA1-related ANSD revealed elongation of eV latencies. Interesting to notice that electrically evoked action potentials were absent in these patients. These finds are in concordance with the pathophysiological mechanism of OPA1-related ANSD, described above. Haploinsofiency of OPA1 protein lead to terminal dendrite dysfunction and pruning, probably therefore action potentials are absent, while spiral ganglion cells themselves are preserve, which is reflected in recordable eABRs. Patients had good speech perception after CI, as it was predicted by eABRs [24].

Despite variation in eABRs in patients with ANSD, there is no universal classification of eABRs wave morphology in patients with ANSD. Kimitaka Kaga, who was one of the first people who described ANSD in a 1994 publication, has proposed to divide eABRs in ANSD into 4 groups. Group A – pre-synaptic ANSD with normal eABR. Group B – pre-synaptic ANSD with abnormal eABR, as in OTOF-related ANSD, elongated eV latency. This elongation is attributed to secondary neurotransmission disorders due to synaptic dysfunction. Group C – EABRs are detected in post-synaptic cases because electric stimulation could bypass the site of lesion. In this group OPA1-related ANSD and other cases of post-synaptic auditory synaptopathy cases eABRs might be included. Group D – absent eABRs in post-synaptic cases. Most demyelinating diseases and "true" auditory neuropathy cases would be included in this group.

When there is no data about the etiology of ANSD distinguishing between groups A, B, and C might be slightly difficult because eV latency might be elongated due to maturational delay in the early period after CI.

According to our experience, the main sign that electrical stimulation bypassed the site of lesion, therefore peripheral hearing deficit in ANSD patients is compensated and good CI outcomes might be expected, is the presence of eABRs (even with slightly elongated wave latency) in monopolar mode stimulation from apical, middle and basal electrodes [51].

6.3 Our experience of eABR testing in children with ANSD

Registration of eABRs was carried out in 25 children with ANSD (CI at the age of 1,5 to 5 years) at different times after cochlear implantation. 8 children were with OTOF-related ANSD, 10 with perinatal risk factors (9 prematurity with or without hyperbilirubinemia and 1 with just hyperbilirubinemia), 2 children with cochlear nerve deficiency (hypoplasia), and 5 children with unknown etiology of ANSD.

EABRS were recorded ipsilaterally, but if stimulus artifacts conceal the response, we used contralateral recordings for eABR analysis. EABRS were measured in monopolar mode, biphasic pulse stimuli with pulse duration 25–100 ms for Cochlear and 75 ms for Advanced Bionics, stimulation rate 25–26 Hz. Measurements were performed at least for three intracochlear electrodes (in basal, middle, and apical turn). If there was no response or responses in monopolar mode were inconclusive, the bipolar mode of stimulation was performed.

The standard stimulation parameters (biphasic stimulus phase width, stimulation rate) were sufficient for a clear registration of eABRs waves (eIII, eV) in all 8 children with OTOF-related ANSD and in all 10 children with perinatal risk factors for ANSD. The presence of eABRs in OTOF-related cases (**Figure 4**) matches the pathophysiology described above, and the wave latencies were elongated just as was described by other researchers [50]. Presence of eABRs in all cases with perinatal risk factors indicates that the main disorders involve inner hair cells in the case of prematurity as it was seen in histological findings [52]. Even in the case of hyperbelirubin-related ANSD, electrical stimulation bypassed the site of lesion. In children with hypoplastic cochlear nerve, EABRs were absent or partially recorded only from basal electrodes with elongated phase width up to 100 ms in monopolar mode and in case of bipolar mode of stimulation of high intensity in basal turn. In children with unknown etiology of ANSD in two cases eABRS were recordable from all stimulated electrodes in monopolar mode, in other three cases eABRs were absent or recordable only from basal electrodes at a high intensity of stimulation and/or in bipolar mode of stimulation in the basal turn of the cochlea. These patients with unknown etiology but recordable robust eABRs probably have auditory synaptopathy type of ANSD, whereas patients with absent or partially recordable eABRs have auditory neuropathy type of ANSD.

Results of rehabilitation after cochlear implantation corresponded to the results of registration of eABRs. There were much better among children with robust eABRs from all tested electrodes in monopolar mode of stimulation. All 5 children with absent or partially recordable eABRs from the basal turn in monopolar or bipolar

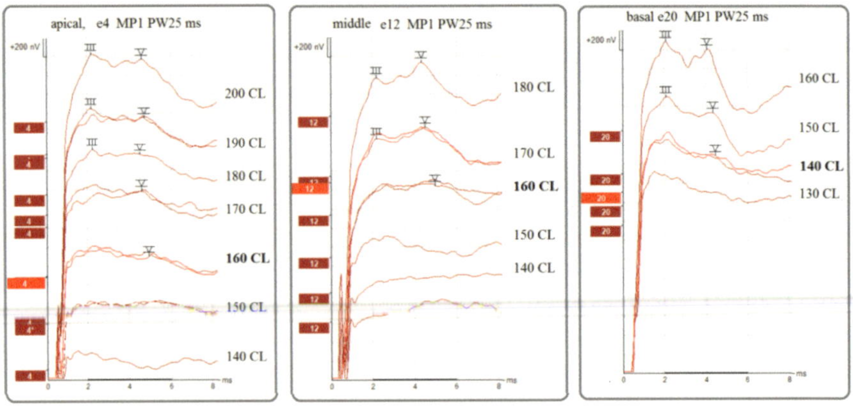

Figure 4.
EABRs from apical, middle, and basal electrodes from a child with OTOF-related ANSD, 1st day after speech processor switch-on.

mode end up with necessity of using sign language for communication. However, the selection of optimal parameters for recording eABRs made it possible to make appropriate changes to the speech processor stimulation map, which improved the perception and some discrimination of sounds. So, these 5 children had some benefit from CI, but not enough for hearing-based communication. The absence of eABRs might help to make a decision about including alternative methods of communication at an earlier stage of rehabilitation.

The thresholds of eABRs were much higher than the thresholds level of patients' speech processor stimulation map and they were closer to the maximum comfortable level of stimulation. Determination of the eABRs thresholds may help to predict the maximum comfortable level of stimulation, which is especially important in small and non-contact patients. However, this statement requires further research.

According to our data, most valuable parameters of eABRs for predicting positive outcomes after CI is recordable eABRs from intracochlear electrodes in basal, middle, and apical turn electrodes in the monopolar mode of stimulation. Latencies of eABRs do not seem to be crucial for rehabilitation outcomes. While absent or partially recordable eABRs indicate that electrical stimulation even if it causes a sound sensation, does not fully bypass the site of the lesion and cannot fully compensate hearing deficit, so an alternative way of communication might be needed.

7. Conclusions

ANSD diagnosis is not a difficult task for modern audiology, but which rehabilitation approach is optimal for the certain child and what rehabilitation outcomes we could hope for – are still quite tricky questions.

Revealing the genetic mechanism of ANSD allows understanding the lesion localization in the auditory system, which in most cases cannot be done using only standard non-invasive audiological examination methods. Identification of the genetic etiology of ANSD is extremely important, as it can make it possible to predict the course of the disease, the appearance of other symptoms in case of syndromic forms, and also to choose the optimal method of rehabilitation based on the localization of the pathology and the pathophysiology of hearing loss.

When the etiology of ANSD is unknown, registration of eABRs immediately after cochlear implantation may allow predicting the maximum rehabilitation potential of a child with ANSD. EABRs help with the choice of optimal patient management tactics, including planning the inclusion of alternative communication methods, as early as possible after cochlear implantation incase of auditory neuropathy type of ANSD.

Author details

Maria Lalayants[1,2]

1 Russian Children's Clinical Hospital of the FSAEI HE RSMU Named after N.I. Pirogov of the Ministry of Health of the Russian Federation, Moscow, Russia

2 Russian Medical Academy of Continuing Professional Education, Moscow, Russia

*Address all correspondence to: layantsmr@yandex.ru

References

[1] Kaga K, Starr A. Neuropathies of the Auditory and Vestibular Eighth Cranial Nerves. Tokyo: Springer; 2009. p. 159. DOI: 10.1007/978-4-431-09433-3

[2] Hayes D, Sininger YS. Guidelines for Identification and Management of Infants and Young Children with Auditory Neuropathy Spectrum Disorder. In: Guidlines development conference at NHS, Como, Italy. 2008. 52 p. Available from: https://www.childrenscolorado.org/globalassets/departments/ear-nose-throat/ansd-monograph.pdf on 04.03.2023

[3] Berlin CI, Hood LJ, Morlet T, Wilensky D, Li L, Mattingly KR, et al. Multi-site diagnosis and management of 260 patients with auditory neuropathy/dys-synchrony (auditory neuropathy spectrum disorder). International Journal of Audiology. 2010;**49**(1):30-43. DOI: 10.3109/14992020903160892

[4] Rajput K, Saeed M, Ahmed J, Chung M, Munro C, Patel S, et al. Findings from aetiological investigation of auditory neuropathy Spectrum disorder in children referred to cochlear implant programs. International Journal of Pediatric Otorhinolaryngology. 2019;**116**:79-83. DOI: 10.1016/j.ijporl.2018.10.010

[5] Saluja S, Agarwal A, Kler N, Amin S. Auditory neuropathy spectrum disorder in late preterm and term infants with severe jaundice. International Journal of Pediatric Otorhinolaryngology. 2010;**74**:1292-1297

[6] Saidia AR, Ruel J, Bahloul A, Chaix B, Venail F, Wang J. Current advances in gene therapies of genetic auditory neuropathy Spectrum disorder. Journal of. Clinical Medicine. 2023;**12**(3):738. [Internet] Available from:. DOI: 10.3390/jcm12030738

[7] Miyagawa M, Nishio SY, Usami SI. A comprehensive study on the etiology of patients receiving cochlear implantation with special emphasis on genetic epidemiology. Otology & Neurotology. 2016;**37**(2):e126

[8] Breneman AI, Gifford RH, Dejong MD. Cochlear implantation in children with auditory neuropathy spectrum disorder: Long-term outcomes. Journal of the American Academy of Audiology. 2012;**23**(1):5-17. DOI: 10.3766/jaaa.23.1.2

[9] Neary W, Lightfoot G. Auditory neuropathy spectrum disorder: Examples of poor progress following cochlear implantation. Audiology Medicine. 2012;**10**:142-149

[10] Shearer AE, Hansen MR. Auditory synaptopathy, auditory neuropathy, and cochlear implantation. Laryngoscope Investigated Otolaryngology. 2019;**4**(4):429-440. DOI: 10.1002/lio2.288

[11] Moser T, Starr A. Auditory neuropathy — Neural and synaptic mechanisms. Nature Reviews. Neurology. 2016;**12**:135-149. DOI: 10.1038/nrneurol.2016.10

[12] Chaudhry D, Chaudhry A, Muzaffar J, Monksfield P, Bance M. Cochlear implantation outcomes in post synaptic auditory neuropathies: A systematic review and narrative synthesis. The Journal of International Advanced Otology. 2020;**16**(3):411-431. DOI: 10.5152/iao.2020.9035

[13] Lin P-H, Wu H-P, Wu C-M, Chiang Y-T, Hsu JS, Tsai C-Y, et al. Cochlear implantation outcomes in patients with auditory neuropathy Spectrum disorder of genetic and non-genetic etiologies: A multicenter

study. Biomedicine. 2022;**10**(7):1523. [Internet] Available from:. DOI: 10.3390/biomedicines10071523

[14] Kim BJ, Jang JH, Han JH, et al. Mutational and phenotypic spectrum of OTOF-related auditory neuropathy in Koreans: Eliciting reciprocal interaction between bench and clinics. Journal of Translational Medicine. 2018;**16**:330. DOI: 10.1186/s12967-018-1708-z

[15] Rodríguez-Ballesteros M, Reynoso R, Olarte M, et al. A multicenter study on the prevalence and spectrum of mutations in the otoferlin gene (OTOF) in subjects with nonsyndromic hearing impairment and auditory neuropathy. Human Mutation. 2008;**29**(6):823-831

[16] Varga R, Avenarius MR, Kelley PM, Keats BJ, Berlin CI, Hood LJ, et al. OTOF mutations revealed by genetic analysis of hearing loss families including a potential temperature sensitive auditory neuropathy allele. Journal of Medical Genetics. 2006;**43**(7):576-581. DOI: 10.1136/jmg.2005.038612

[17] Wu CC, Hsu CJ, Huang FL, Lin YH, Lin YH, Liu TC, et al. Timing of cochlear implantation in auditory neuropathy patients with OTOF mutations: Our experience with 10 patients. Clinical Otolaryngology. 2018;**43**:352-357

[18] Santarelli R, del Castillo I, Cama E, Scimemi P, Starr A. Audibility, speech perception and processing of temporal cues in ribbon synaptic disorders due to OTOF mutations. Hearing Research. 2015;**330**(pt B):200-212

[19] Ruel J, Emery S, Nouvian R, Bersot T, Amilhon B, Van Rybroek JM, et al. Impairment of SLC17A8 encoding vesicular glutamate transporter-3, VGLUT3, underlies nonsyndromic deafness DFNA25 and inner hair cell dysfunction in null mice. American Journal of Human Genetics. 2008;**83**(2):278-292. DOI: 10.1016/j.ajhg.2008.07.008

[20] Baig SM, Koschak A, Lieb A, et al. Loss of Ca(v)1.3 (CACNA1D) function in a human channelopathy with bradycardia and congenital deafness. Nature Neuroscience. 2011;**14**(1):77-84

[21] Brandt A, Striessnig J, Moser T. CaV1.3 channels are essential for development and presynaptic activity of cochlear inner hair cells. The Journal of Neuroscience. 2003;**23**(34):10832-10840

[22] Schrauwen I, Helfmann S, Inagaki A, et al. A mutation in CABP2, expressed in cochlear hair cells, causes autosomal-recessive hearing impairment. American Journal of Human Genetics. 2012;**91**(4):636-645

[23] Huang T, Santarelli R, Starr A. Mutation of OPA1 gene causes deafness by affecting function of auditory nerve terminals. Brain Research. 2009;**1300**:97-104. DOI: 10.1016/j.brainres.2009.08.083 Epub 2009 Sep 3

[24] Santarelli R, Rossi R, Scimemi P, Cama E, Valentino ML, La Morgia C, et al. OPA1-related auditory neuropathy: Site of lesion and outcome of cochlear implantation. Brain. 2015;**138**(Pt 3):563-576. DOI: 10.1093/brain/awu378 Epub 2015 Jan 5

[25] Schoen CJ, Emery SB, Thorne MC, Ammana HR, Sliwerska E, Arnett J, et al. Increased activity of diaphanous homolog 3 (DIAPH3)/diaphanous causes hearing defects in humans with auditory neuropathy and in drosophila. Proceedings of the National Academy of Sciences of the United States of America. 2010;**107**(30):13396-13401. DOI: 10.1073/pnas.1003027107 Epub 2010 Jul 12

[26] Han K-H, Oh D-Y, Lee S, et al. ATP1A3 mutations can cause progressive

auditory neuropathy: A new gene of auditory synaptopathy. Scientific Reports. 2017;**7**(1):1-11

[27] Ćeranić B, Luxon LM. Progressive auditory neuropathy in patients with Leber's hereditary optic neuropathy. Journal of Neurology, Neurosurgery & Psychiatry. 2004;**75**:626-630. DOI: 10.1136/jnnp.2003.017673

[28] Lerat J, Magdelaine C, Roux A, Darnaud L, Beauvais-Dzugan H, Naud S, et al. Hearing loss in inherited peripheral neuropathies: Molecular diagnosis by NGS in a French series. Molecular Genetics & Genomic Medicine. 2019;**7**(9):e839. DOI: 10.1002/mgg3.839. Available from: https://onlinelibrary.wiley.com

[29] Butinar D, Starr A, Zidar J, et al. Auditory nerve is affected in one of two different point mutations of the neurofi lament light gene. Clinical Neurophysiology. 2008;**119**:367-375

[30] Starr A, Michalewski HJ, Zeng F-G, et al. Pathology and physiology of auditory neuropathy with a novel mutation in the MPZ gene (Tyr145->Ser). Brain. 2003;**126**(pt 7):1604-1619

[31] Seeman P, Mazanec R, Huehne K, Suslíková P, Keller O, Rautenstrauss B. Hearing loss as the first feature of late-onset axonal CMT disease due to a novel P0 mutation. Neurology. 2004;**63**(4):733-735. DOI: 10.1212/01.wnl.0000134605.61307.de

[32] Verhagen WI, Huygen PL, Gabreëls-Festen AA, Engelhart M, van Mierlo PJ, van Engelen BG. Sensorineural hearing impairment in patients with Pmp22 duplication, deletion, and frameshift mutations. Otology & Neurotology. 2005;**26**(3):405-414. DOI: 10.1097/01.mao.0000169769.93173.df

[33] Anzalone CL, Nuhanovic S, Olund AP, Carlson ML. Cochlear implantation in Charcot-Marie-tooth disease: Case report and review of the literature. Case Reports in Medicine. 2018;**2018**:1760978. DOI: 10.1155/2018/1760978

[34] Rance G, Corben L, Delatycki M. Auditory processing deficits in children with Friedreich ataxia. Journal of Child Neurology. 2012;**27**(9):1197-1203. DOI: 10.1177/0883073812448963

[35] Karzon R, Narayanan A, Chen L, Judith E, Lieu C. Tamara Hershey longitudinal hearing loss in Wolfram syndrome. Orphanet Journal of Rare Diseases. 2018;**13**:102. DOI: 10.1186/s13023-018-0852-0

[36] Cif L, Gonzalez V, Garcia-Ptacek S, et al. Progressive dystonia in Mohr-Tranebjaerg syndrome with cochlear implant and deep brain stimulation. Movement Disorders. 2013;**28**(6):737-738. DOI: 10.1002/mds.25519

[37] Zong L, Guan J, Ealy M, et al. Mutations in apoptosis-inducing factor cause X-linked recessive auditory neuropathy spectrum disorder. Journal of Medical Genetics. 2015;**52**(8):523-531. DOI: 10.1136/jmedgenet-2014-102961

[38] Simon M, Richard EM, Wang X, et al. Mutations of human NARS2, encoding the mitochondrial asparaginyl-tRNA synthetase, cause nonsyndromic deafness and Leigh syndrome. PLoS Genetics. 2015;**11**(3):e1005097. Published 2015 Mar 25. DOI: 10.1371/journal.pgen.1005097

[39] Feng B, Jin C, Cheng Z, Zhao X, Sun Z, Zheng X, et al. Mitochondrial dysfunction and therapeutic targets in auditory neuropathy. Neural Plasticity. 2020;**2020**:8843485. DOI: 10.1155/2020/8843485

[40] Tufatulin GS, Koroleva IV, Mefodovskaya EK, Garbaruk ES,

Levin SV, Sugarova SB, et al. Auditory neuropathy case in the child TWNK gene mutations. Innovation technology in hearing loss testing and rehabilitation of patients with hearing loss and deafness. Moscow Conference materials. 2022. p. 62-63 [in Russ]

[41] Jeon JH, Bae MR, Song MH, Noh SH, Choi KH, Choi JY. Relationship between electrically evoked auditory brainstem response and auditory performance after cochlear implant in patients with auditory neuropathy spectrum disorder. Otology & Neurotology. 2013;**34**(7):1261-1266. DOI: 10.1097/mao.0b013e318291c632

[42] User Guide for eABR Test Procedure. Eclipse with CI systems. www.Interacoustics.com

[43] Cochlear Clinical Guidance Document. 2010. www.Coclear.com

[44] Dziemba OC, Hocke T, Müller A, Kaftan H. Excitation characteristic of a bipolar stimulus for broadband stimulation in measurements of electrically evoked auditory potentials. Zeitschrift fur Medizinische Physik. 2018;**28**(1):73-77. DOI: 10.1016/j.zemedi.2017.09.008

[45] Kaga K. ABRs and electrically evoked ABRs in children. In: Modern Otology and Neurotology. Tokyo: Springer; 2022. DOI: 10.1007/978-4-431-54189-9_1

[46] Hughes ML. Objective Measures in Cochlear Implants. San Diego: Plural Pub; 2013

[47] Gordon KA, Papsin BC, Harrison RV. Activity-dependent developmental plasticity of the auditory brain stem in children who use cochlear implants. Ear and Hearing. 2003;**24**(6):485-500. DOI: 10.1097/01.aud.0000100203.65990.d4

[48] Shallop JK, Peterson A, Facer GW, Fabry LB, Driscoll CL. Cochlear implants in five cases of auditory neuropathy: Postoperative findings and progress. The Laryngoscope. 2001;**111**(4 Pt 1):555-562. DOI: 10.1097/00005537-200104000-00001

[49] Runge-Samuelson CL, Drake S, Wackym PA. Quantitative analysis of electrically evoked auditory brainstem responses in implanted children with auditory neuropathy/dyssynchrony. Otology & Neurotology. 2008;**29**(2):174-178. DOI: 10.1097/mao.0b013e31815aee4b

[50] Hosoya M. et al. Elongated EABR wave latencies observed in patients with auditory neuropathy caused by OTOF mutation //Laryngoscope Investigative Otolaryngology. – 2018. – T. 3. – №. 5. – C. 388-393

[51] Lalayants MR, Chugunova TI, Bakhshinyan VV, Tavartkiladze GA. Electrically evoked ABR through cochlear implant in children with auditory neuropathy spectrum disorder. Vestnik Oto-Rino-Laringologii. 2022;**87**(2):4-9. DOI: 10.17116/otorino2022870214 [In Russ]

[52] Amatuzzi M, Liberman MC, Northrop C. Selective inner hair cell loss in prematurity: A temporal bone study of infants from a neonatal intensive care unit. Journal of the Association for Research in Otolaryngology. 2011;**12**(5):595-604. DOI: 10.1007/s10162-011-0273-4. Epub 2011 Jun 14